Excerpts from
The MEDICAL and NUTRITIONAL APPROACH To
PROSTATE PROBLEMS

The Prostate is often referred to as the *"male motor"* or *"sexual brain."* Prostate problems occur in men over 40.   Chapter 1

* * *

It is the prostate gland that is essential for the swift thrust of semen during intercourse and aids in the climax experience.   Chapter 2

* * *

Uncontrolled dripping from the penis and the feeling of incomplete emptying of the bladder can indicate acute prostatitis. Too much sex stimulation without release is sometimes the cause.   Chapter 3

* * *

A decrease in the force or size of the stream when urinating may indicate an enlarged prostate. If not taken care of, such a condition could lead to bladder or kidney stones.   Chapter 6

* * *

There are **four** types of surgery for Cancer of the prostate. Such surgery may leave you impotent, unable to have intercourse. Chapter 8

* * *

Some nutritionists suggest that both zinc and bee pollen are highly effective in preventing an enlarged prostate.

* * *

There are **3** enemies to a healthy prostate gland. Some believe a series of cleansing enemas provides helpful relief.   Chapter 11

* * *

The early stages of prostate problems may begin with a dull, aching pain in the nape of the neck. There may also be a loss of sex drive or the inability to maintain an erection.   Chapter 12

* * *

Several types of sexual practices are hard on the prostate gland and eventually the multiple problems of an enlarged prostate follow. If one understands the function of the prostate it is the first step towards a happy and healthy sexual life.   Chapter 13

* * *

All this and <u>much more</u> you will find in the chapters of this revealing book on *The Medical Approach versus The Nutritional Approach To Prostate Problems!*

Important Legal Notice

The Medical Approach versus The Nutritional Approach To **PROSTATE PROBLEMS**

by Salem Kirban

Published by SALEM KIRBAN, Inc., Kent Road, Huntingdon Valley, Pennsylvania 19006. Copyright © 1982 by Salem Kirban. Printed in United States of America. All rights reserved, including the right to reproduce this book or portions thereof in any form.

Library of Congress Catalog Card No. 81-84442
ISBN 0-912582-46-4

ACKNOWLEDGMENTS

To **Estelle Bair Composition** for excellence in typesetting.

To **Walter W. Slotilock,** Chapel Hill Litho, for negatives.

To **Bob Jackson,** for illustrations on pages 14, 20, 24, 25, 31, 33, 34, 36, 39, 40, 44.

To **Dickinson Brothers, Inc.,** for printing this book.

And special thanks to the following publishers for graciously making available medical illustrations for this book:

Intermed Communications, Inc., Springhouse, Pennsylvania 19477
Illustrations reprinted with permission from Diseases, Copyright © 1981.

J.B. Lippincott Company, Philadelphia, Pennsylvania 19105
Illustrations reprinted with permission from Textbook of Medical-Surgical Nursing by L. Brunner and D. Suddarth, ed. 4, Copyright © 1980.

Mitchell Beazley Publishers, Ltd., England
Atlas of the Body and Mind, Copyright © Mitchell Beazley Publishers, Ltd. 1976. Published in U.S.A. by **Rand McNally & Company.**

CONTENTS

Special Features Include

Bibliography
Recommended Reading

Airola, Paavo, *How To Get Well,* Health Plus Publishers, Phoenix, Arizona, 1976.

Biser, Sam, *Healthview Newsletter,* Nos. 15, 16, Charlottesville, Virginia 22901.

Cooley, Donald G., Better Homes and Gardens *After-40 Health and Medical Guide,* Meredith Corporation, Des Moines, Iowa 1980.

Kolodny, Masters, William H., Johnson, Virginia E., *Textbook of Sexual Medicine,* Little, Brown and Company, Boston, 1979.

Nourse, Alan E., M.D., *Ladies' Home Journal Family Medical Guide,* Harper & Row, New York, 1973.

Rothenberg, Robert E., M.D., *The Complete Surgical Guide,* Weathervane Books, New York, 1974.

Tobe, John H., *Your Prostate: Treatment and Prevention,* Provoker Press, St. Catharines, Ontario, Canada, 1968.

Troy, Marian T., *Better Bowel Health,* Pyramid Books, New York, 1974.

1

PROSTATE . . . THE SEXUAL MOTOR

There are many definitions for the Prostate. It has been called *"the male motor."* It has also been referred to as *"the sexual brain."*

Prostate problems are <u>not</u> selective in that they affect both the rich, the middle class and the poor as well as the well-known and the worker. Prostate problems <u>are</u> selective in that it is a disease which occurs in men only and after the age of 40. Do not confuse the word prostrate with the male gland, the pro<u>state</u>!

Women do **not** have a prostate gland so they are not affected by diseases of the prostate.

At 76, the motion picture actor, Henry Fonda was fighting a battle both with heart disease and cancer of the prostate.

Next to lung cancer, prostatic cancer has the highest incidence of any form of male cancer. About 57,000 new cases are diagnosed in the United States each year. More than 20,000 American males die of the disease every year!

MALE Reproductive System

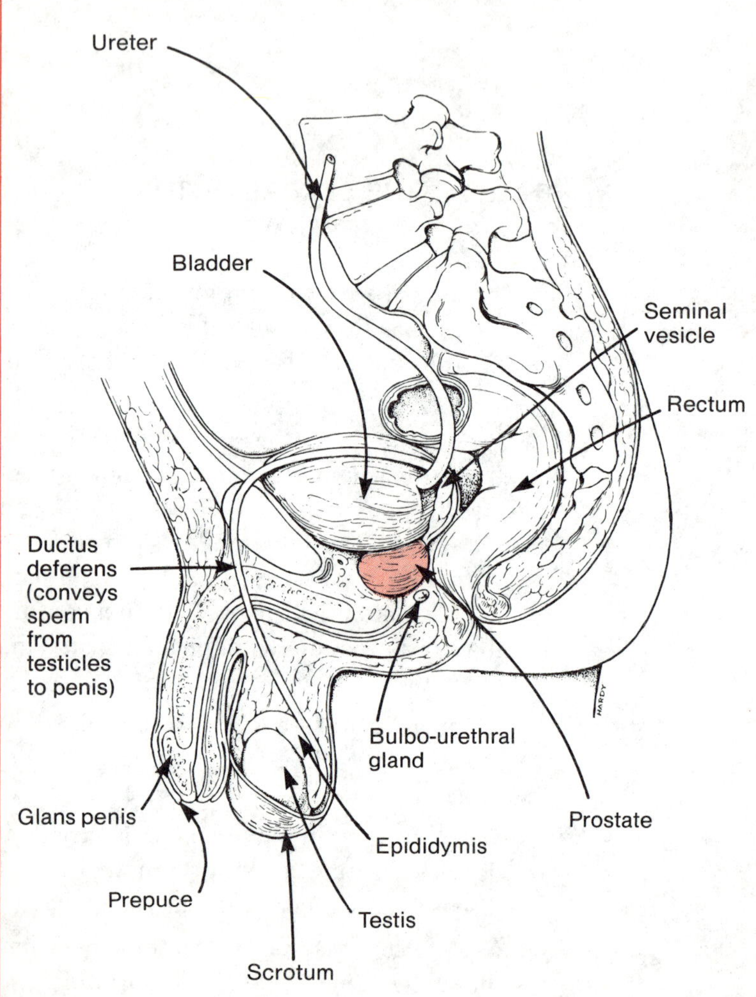

Illustration courtesy J. B. Lipincott Company (from Chaffee, E. E., and Greisheimer, E.M.: Basic Physiology and Anatomy, 3rd ed., Philadelphia, 1974).

PROSTATE CHARACTERISTICS

Prostate . . .
Part Glandular
Part Muscular

The prostate is a male genital gland about the size of a chestnut. It lies just below the urinary bladder and surrounds the first inch of the urethra, the canal that carries urine from the bladder.

The prostate is partly glandular and partly muscular. About 1/4th of the prostate is made up of glandular tissue. The prostate is about 1½ inches in its three dimensions and weighs about 1 ounce. The gland has three main ducts (lobes) that open into the urethra.

The urethra discharges urine through the penis at the outlet of the bladder (which is called the _posterior urethra_).

The _anterior urethra_ is found on the shaft of the penis. _Posterior_ means _back_ and _anterior_ means _front_.

PROSTATE CAN BLOCK BLADDER

Prostate
Encircles
Urethra

The prostate gland encircles the urethra. And the urethra is the channel through which urine passes from the bladder to the penis. One can see if the prostate becomes enlarged it will squeeze the urinary channel and cause either partial or complete obstruction of the bladder. This inability to urinate completely is a problem common in older men. And it can cause further complications.

PROSTATE FUNCTIONS

The prostate has several functions:

1. It stores the sperm
2. It produces seminal fluid
3. It controls the muscles that allows you to urinate
4. It controls the muscles that trigger you to ejaculate

The testicles *(testes)* manufacture the spermatozoa. This is then passed to the prostate gland. It takes over, adding its own fluids, which contain several vital substances. One substance the prostate produces is a waxlike material which coats the sperm so that it can survive in the otherwise lethal high acidity of the vagina.

Provides Sperm Fluid

Sperm in the Greek means _seed_. Sperm is a milky, opalescent fluid. It has a distinctive smell which comes from the prostate fluid. About 40% of the male's ejaculation is thin, milky fluid released by the prostate. This fluid provides the medium in which the sperm will swim. Then comes the sperm themselves (from 150-400 million) and finally both the seminal vesicles and the prostate release a sticky yellow fluid. This acts as a food supply for the sperm on their journey. The sperm represent only about 2% of the seminal fluid.

The seminal fluid is produced continuously at about 5-30 drops an hour. During sexual excitement production is increased. If there is an overflow of fluid it is discharged a little at a time in the urine.

2

THE PROSTATE SEXUAL FUNCTION

PROSTATE DURING SEX

To properly understand the functions of the prostate one should be aware of the bodily interactions that occur during sexual intercourse.

Active in Coitus

Sexual intercourse is termed *coitus*. Coitus means *to go together*.

Sexual intercourse is the insertion of the penis (the male organ) into the vagina (the female organ) during sexual arousal. The insertion of the penis brings about increasing sexual excitement until a climax (*orgasm*) is reached. Orgasm is described as a swelling or fullness and is an overwhelming intense feeling of pleasure. This is centered on the genital area primarily.

Prostate . . . Important In Sexual Relations

During sexual intercourse the heartbeat increases to twice the normal rate. As the climax approaches, an automatic series of muscular contractions occur around the urethra and prostate. This brings about three or four bursts of semen at intervals of about 1 second apart. The prostate exercises such ejaculatory force that the semen can be propelled from a few inches to a few feet. At this point the penis is about 1½ times its normal size but slowly reduces to normal after ejaculation. The amount of ejaculation averages a small teaspoonful.

The man has his <u>orgasm</u> at the point of ejaculation of semen. The woman goes through the same pleasurable stages. However, she takes longer to reach her plateau and can maintain it at a higher level for longer.[1]

Rather than the semen simply flowing into the uterus, the prostate muscles contract and pump the stored fluid along with the sperm and other secretions.

THE MALE SEXUAL MOTOR

The Explosive Expeller!

The ejaculation has several purposes:

1. Prevents semen from remaining in the urethra and coagulating.
2. Buckshot-type thrust of semen better insures it penetrating the uterus.
3. Climactic ejaculation makes the male somewhat immobile. This prevents him from withdrawing in an attempt to defeat nature's purpose.

[1]For a complete study of the sexual act, send for <u>The Medical Approach versus The Nutritional Approach To IMPOTENCE/FRIGIDITY</u> by Salem Kirban. Send $6 ($1 is for postage) to: Salem Kirban, Inc., Kent Road, Huntingdon Valley, Pennsylvania 19006.

The prostate is a vital organ in the male and provides for him sexual gratification as well as the desire. The prostate with its powerful muscular action during intercourse can truly be called the "*male sexual motor.*"

Releases Hormones

Not only does the prostate store fluid which is pumped out during intercourse but it also makes and releases hormones. The prostate is perhaps the most important and least understood of all sexual organs in the male.

PROSTATE PLAYS IMPORTANT ROLE

Understanding The Bladder Function

In understanding the prostate it is also important to understand the function of the bladder. The bladder is an expandable sac. It is constructed of layers of smooth muscle and is sensitive to stretching. When accumulated urine fills the bladder, the individual becomes aware of a progressive discomfort until the bladder is emptied. An average of 1½ quarts of urine is secreted in a 24-hour period. If less than one pint of urine is secreted (voided) in a 24-hour period it could be a sign of impaired kidney function. If more than 2 quarts are secreted, it could indicate diabetes or pituitary gland disease.

During urination, the urine is passed from the bladder through another tube, the urethra, to the outside.

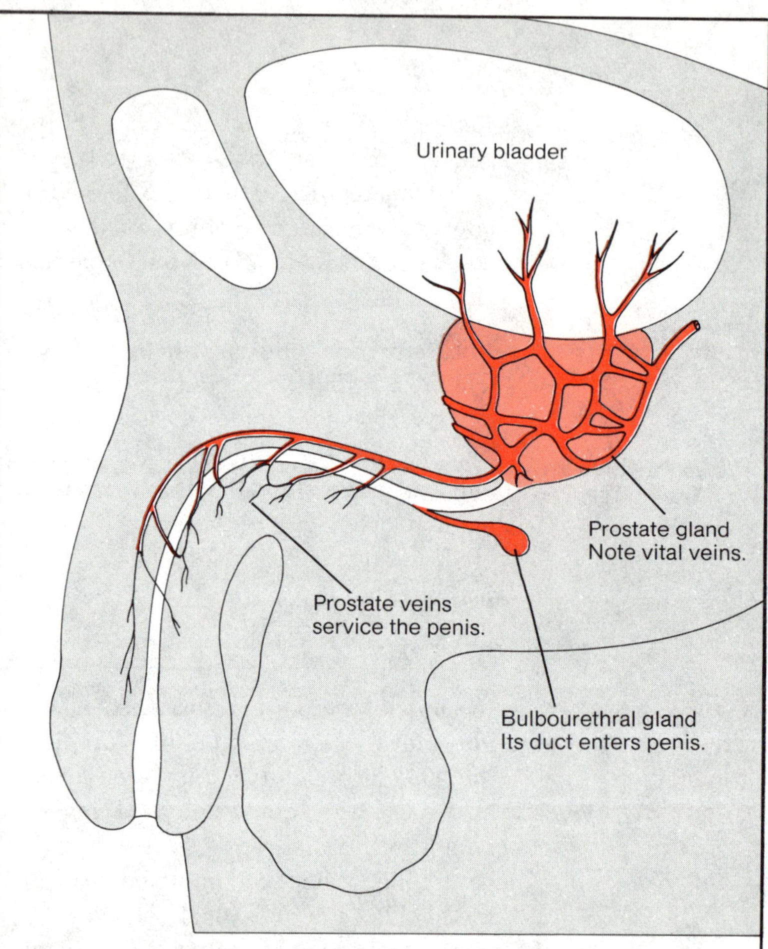

Illustration shows rich vein structure enveloping the Prostate gland. One can see how an enlarged prostate would cause problems in the urinary system. It is the rhythmic contractions of the prostate that play an important part in ejaculation during sexual intercourse.

The Prostate gland produces a clear alkaline fluid that becomes part of the seminal ejaculation fluid. The Prostate gland also is a major site for the synthesis of <u>prostaglandins</u>. The prostaglandins affect the heart and smooth muscles. The <u>Bulbourethral glands</u> secrete a fluid as well which form part of the seminal fluid. These two small glands are about the size of a pea and are on each side of the Prostate.

While the urethra tube in the female is less than 2 inches long, the urethra tube in the male is much longer (about 6½″). And some 1½″ of it passes directly through the <u>prostate</u> gland soon after leaving the bladder. This segment is sometimes referred to as the <u>*prostatic urethra*</u>. It then passes through the length of the penis to the opening at the tip.

Urine Force Varies

The force of urine is much greater in the child than in the adult because the bladder is more nearly an abdominal than pelvic organ in the child. Thus the abdominal muscles help to expel the urine in the child.

It is unwise to have sexual intercourse when your bladder needs emptying.

Prostate Affects Ejaculation

A weak or poorly functioning prostate can give rise to premature ejaculation, called <u>*coitus praecox*</u>. <u>Praecox</u> means <u>*early*</u>.

When a man has a healthy prostate he has an air of assurance. When suddenly he discovers that his prostate gland is not functioning properly, it can affect his outlook on life. And yet this is the critical time in his life when he should approach each day in a positive, happy manner for:

> *A merry heart*
> *doeth good like medicine:*
> *but a broken spirit*
> *drieth the bones.*
>
> (Proverbs 17:22)

Sexual Functions Of Prostate

Some have said that a man's virility (his sexual power) is a vital link to his accomplishments. The more potent a man is sexually, the greater is the drive within him. If this is true, one can see why a malfunctioning prostate can be a source of real concern to a man.

The prostate in sexual intercourse:

1. Activates the seminal fluid.
2. Assists in the erection and maintaining the erection of the penis.
3. Helps provide lubricating fluid for the sex act.
4. Produces the power for the ejaculation during the act of intercourse.
5. Helps control both the <u>duration</u> and the <u>frequency</u> of the sexual act.

A Versatile Organ

The prostate also plays an important function with the bladder in controlling the flow of urine.

The prostate, it would appear, is like a busy airline terminal like Chicago or Atlanta. The prostate, filled with nerve fibre and a concentration of blood is called upon in short notice to prepare the seminal flow and ejaculate. Like an air control tower, it somehow signals a switch at regular intervals to bring about a desire for sexual relations. Then, at several times during the day it must open and shut valves to allow for passage of urine.

3

WHEN THE PROSTATE PROTESTS

PROSTATE ILLS THAT CAN OCCUR

As men grow older, instead of performing heroic functions, the prostate tends to become the General of Malfunctions! Let's look at some problems that can occur.

1. Prostatitis (Acute and Chronic)
2. Prostatism (Enlarged Prostate)
3. Cancer of the Prostate

PROSTATITIS (ACUTE)

Acute Prostatitis is a common ailment that affects men from young adulthood on. It is a bacterial infection of the prostate gland.

The symptoms may develop slowly but acute prostatitis is characterized by the rather abrupt onset of fever. There is also pain at the base of the penis and painful urination. There may be uncontrolled dripping of cloudy fluid from the urethra through the penis. One might feel an incomplete emptying of the bladder. Chills and fever are also a clue to acute prostatitis.

It frequently occurs in young men from 20 to 35. It can be a problem associated with some venereal diseases as well.

The Prostate And Sex

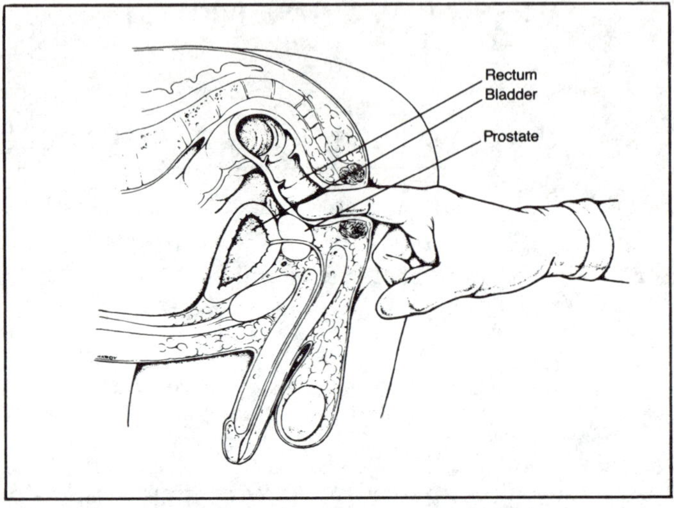

Illustration courtesy J.B. Lippincott Company: Brunner, L., Suddarth, D.: Textbook of Medical-Surgical Nursing. ed. 4, 1980, Philadelphia, J.B. Lippincott.

About 35% of men over age 50 have <u>chronic prostatitis.</u> Low back pain, frequent and urgent urination and painful ejaculation are some of the indicators of this problem. <u>Prostate cancer</u> is the second most common cancer found in men over age 50. Unexplained cystitis, difficulty in starting urinary stream, dribbling, urine retention are possible indicators of prostate cancer. The rectal examination is an essential part of a physical check-up for all men over 40.

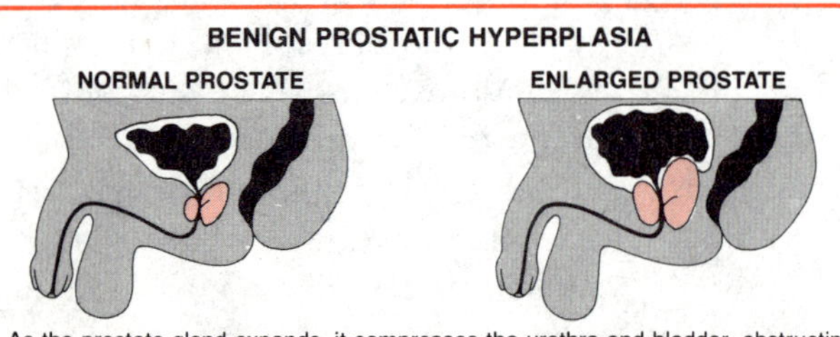

As the prostate gland expands, it compresses the urethra and bladder, obstructing urinary flow.

Illustration reprinted with permission from Diseases, copyright © 1981, Intermed Communications, Inc.

PROSTATIS (CHRONIC)

**A
Nagging
Problem**

Chronic prostatitis can be a more diffi-cult problem because, often, no bacteria can be identified as the certain cause. In chronic prostatitis there is usually no fever but a great frequency of urination. There is loss of libido (*desire for sexual intercourse*). There may also be times when the man is impotent (*inability to ejaculate sperm*).

Some doctors believe that emotions can play a part in chronic prostatitis.

> Caffeine-containing beverages, de-creased sexual activity, prolonged sitting, and many other factors have been associated in popular myth with prostate infections, but scientific evidence does not support these as significant causes.[1]

PROSTATISM
(Benign Prostatic Hypertrophy)

**The
Enlarged
Prostate**

Hypertrophy means *an increase in the size of an organ which does not involve tumor formation.* Thus, in prostatism, the prostate is enlarged. Because the symptoms are somewhat similar, it is often confused with prostatitis.

However, prostatism is a gradual noninfec-tious, noncancerous enlargement of the prostate gland. The problem may not

---

[1]G. Timothy Johnson, M.D. and Stephen E. Goldf-inger, M.D., Health Letter Book (Cambridge, Massachusetts: Harvard University Press) 1981, p. 382.

Night Time Urination A Sign!

evidence itself for many years and when the symptoms start, they may be almost unnoticeable. There may be a tendency to drain a little urine after urination seems complete. One may experience _nocturia,_ the necessity to urinate two or three times or more at night.

Symptoms include:

> Pain in the prostate region
> Discomfort in sitting
> Urgent, painful, burning urination
> Stream of urine that is feeble
>   and dribbles
> Pain during ejaculation at intercourse
> Unexplained bouts of impotence
> Premature ejaculation
> Low back pain

When the prostate increases in size, it can disturb the function of the urethra.

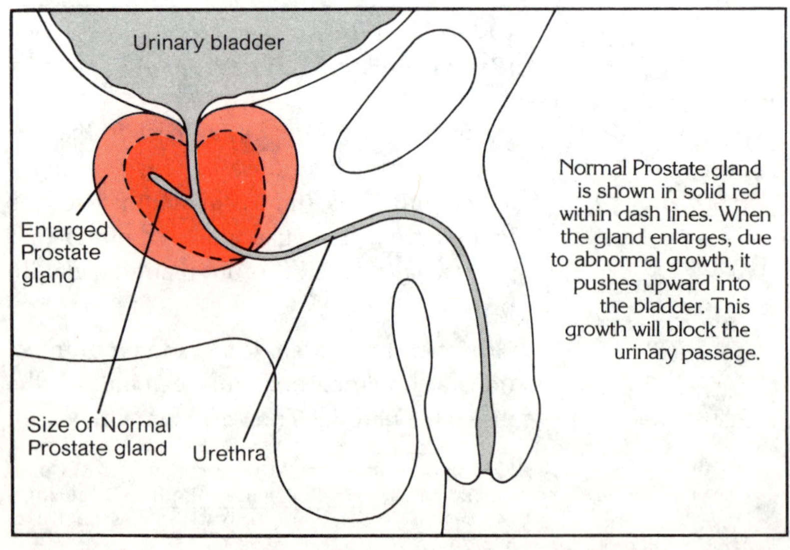

Because the prostate gland surrounds the urethra . . . one can see, as it enlarges, it would narrow the passageway for the urine to flow.

Too Much Sex Stimulation

There are some that believe that prostatism (enlarged prostate) often has its roots in youth. This is the time when sex stimulation is high and relief is low.

> Petting, for example,
> overextends sexual tension
>   without normal release
>   within a reasonable time,
> thus keeping the prostate
>   in an overworked state
>   for too long and too often.

> Continence (*self-restraint*)
> may be even more injurious to the
>   prostate.
> The manufactured sperm is retained
>   with no place to go,
>   putting an additional burden
>   on that gland.

> This concept
> has not been fully accepted
> by the medical profession.[1]

For some reason not precisely known, the prostate begins to enlarge at about age 40. About two out of every three men over 60 have some degree of prostatic enlargement. Enlargement may be caused by some hormone relationship.

When Urine Backs Up!

Sufficiently enlarged, the prostate can make it impossible for the bladder to empty fully. Kidney or bladder stones or infection

---

[1] Sigmund S. Miller, Symptoms (New York: Avon Books) 1978, p. 428.

may result. Urine that is under pressure in the bladder may back up into the kidneys. This causes a condition called _hydrone-phrosis_ which can severely damage kidney function.

The late John H. Tobe, nutritionist and author, described his own prostate problems as follows:

> _Through the years of my life_
> _I have faced worries and troubles_
> _of many kinds and sorts, including_
>   _financial_
>   _marital_
>   _familial as well as others_
> _to which most human beings are subject,_
> _but until I had trouble_
>   _with my prostate,_
> _I must admit that I didn't know_
> _what worry really meant._[1]

John Tobe believed that an enlarged prostate may be caused by a deficiency of Vitamin F. This will be discussed further on in this book.

Continued Erection Problem

There is a condition called _priapism_ (inflammation) which can be caused by prostate disease. It can also be caused by gonorrhea and is sometimes seen in patients with acute leukemia. The penis remains erect even though sexual desire is lacking. The blood rushes into the penis flooding the erectile tissue. If the penis is run under cold water, the erection may subside. Otherwise medical treatment is required.

---

[1]John H. Tobe, Your Prostate, Treatment and Prevention (St. Catharines, Ontario, Canada: Provoker Press) 1968, p. 20.

4

CANCER OF THE PROSTATE

Rectal Examination Important

Cancer of the prostate is one of the major causes of cancer deaths in men . . . about 20,000 per year in the United States. Doctors recommend annual rectal examinations in males over age 50 so that this disease can be detected in its early stages. Most prostate cancers occur in the rear part of the prostate gland. And this can easily be felt during a rectal examination.

The glandular tissue of the prostate resembles that of a woman's breast. Some believe that the cancers are similar. The symptoms of cancer of the prostate are somewhat similar to those of an enlarged prostate. It is identified by the doctor because of the hard, irregular lumps that can be felt during a rectal exam.

If not treated, the disease can spread to other areas of the body such as the bone of the pelvis or the spine. A rise in the level of the enzyme *acid phosphatase* in the serum may indicate cancer of the prostate.

SIGMOIDOSCOPY

A sigmoidoscope is an instrument about 10 inches long. It allows direct visualization of the entire rectum and the lower portion of the large bowel *(the sigmoid).*

This hollow tube (the sigmoidoscope) is lighted. This enables the physician to note any inflammation or tumor growth. He will also be able to remove such polyps or burn them with an electric current. he can also use this instrument to take a biopsy.

Sigmoidoscopy is not a painful procedure. It is generally carried out in a doctor's office without anesthesia. The procedure may be slightly uncomfortable and embarrassing. It is best to have a cleansing enema an hour or two before the procedure. Otherwise, the physician will administer a Fleet-type enema about 15 minutes before he performs the sigmoidoscopy. Some doctors prefer that an enema not be used as the liquid residue may obscure proper vision.

After the sigmoidoscope is lubricated, it is introduced into the rectum, the physician depresses the bellows *(see illustration)* ⟶ to introduce air into the rectum so it is fully expanded for examination. The procedure takes about 10 minutes.

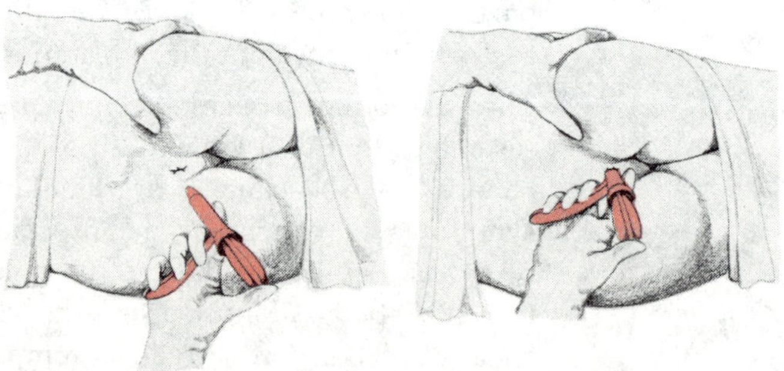

A **<u>proctoscope</u>** is an instrument for inspection of the rectum. In a proctoscope examination, the presence of blood, pus or mucus is observed as well as the mucous membrane. The proctoscope can identify a threadworm infection (commonly known as <u>pinworms</u>). Such an examination is also used to identify internal hemorrhoids.

EXAMINATION OF COLON

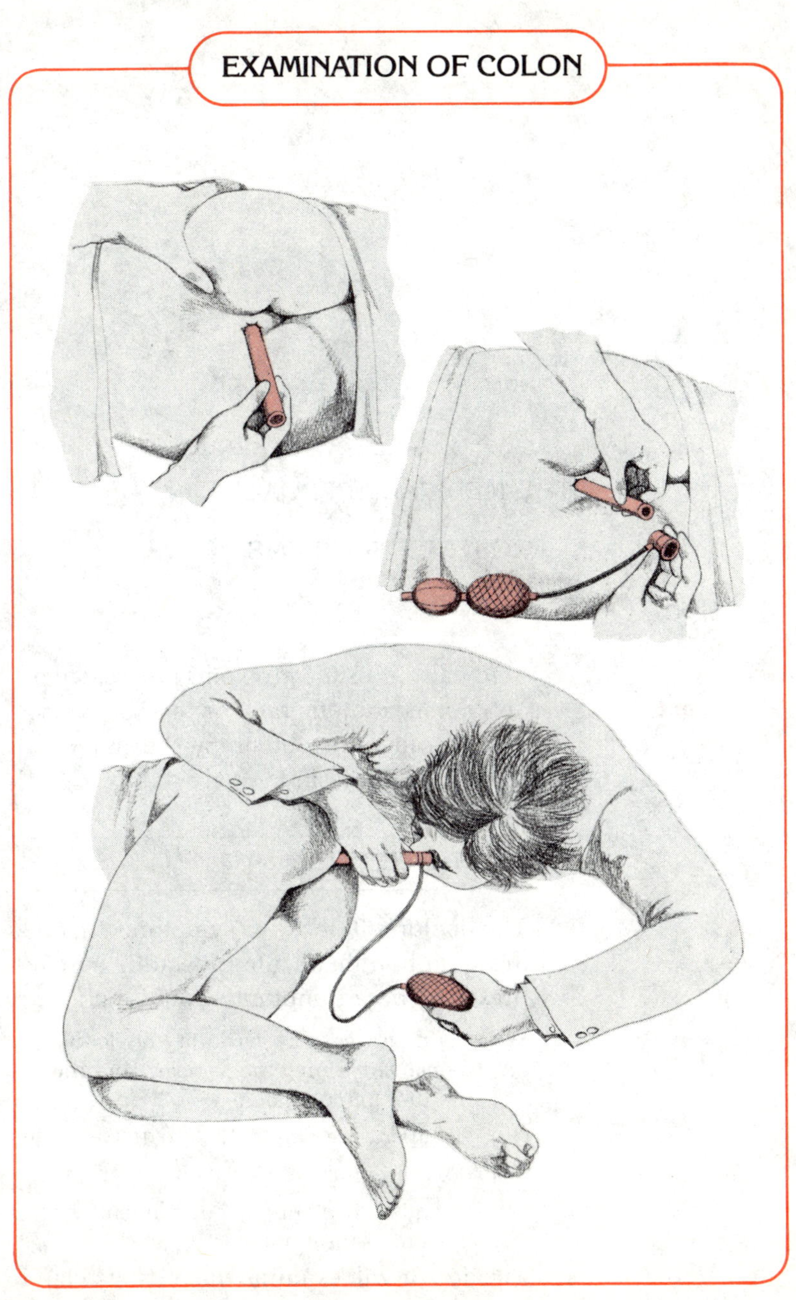

5

THE MEDICAL APPROACH
TO
PROSTATE PROBLEMS

Medically, prostate problems are treated by antibiotics, radiotherapy or radioactive cobalt therapy, chemotherapy, hormone injections, and by surgery.

PROSTATITIS (Acute)

The doctor will look for symptoms that indicate to him that acute prostatitis may be present. These symptoms would include:

1. Pain between the scrotum *(the double pouch containing the testicles)* and the rectum *(the perineum)*.
2. Temperature rise to 101° to 103° F.
3. Pus in the urine.
4. Frequent urination accompanied by a burning sensation.

The doctor will examine the prostate gland

by inserting a gloved finger into the rectum to check on swelling and tenderness.

4 Areas Of Treatment

He may recommend four different avenues of treatment:

1. Bed rest
2. Frequent hot sitz baths daily
3. Drinking large quantities of fluids (like cranberry juice) to flush out the bladder and keep the urine diluted. This also is to avoid the prescribed sulfa drugs from building up in your system.
4. Administration of antibiotic or sulfa drugs

Treatment can continue for two to six weeks. It is usually recommended that you refrain from sexual intercourse until the infection has been eliminated. This may be about six weeks. With acute prostatitis, (in initial stage), rectal massage of the prostate is <u>not</u> advised as it may worsen the inflammation and spread the infection.

PROSTATITIS (CHRONIC)

Pain In Back

One can have <u>chronic</u> prostatitis without ever having acute prostatitis. The most frequent symptoms of <u>chronic</u> prostatitis are:

1. Frequent urination accompanied by a burning sensation
2. Pain in the bladder region or lower part of the back

Medically, treatment of chronic prostatitis

is limited primarily to:

Vigorous Massage

1. Vigorous prostatic massage weekly to promote drainage. This is done by your doctor, and it is best done by a physician who specializes in diseases of the genital organs. Such a physician is called a _urologist_.
2. Drugs such as sulfa combinations. Drugs, however, are not highly successful for this condition.

Medical Times reports:

*Medical treatment
of chronic bacterial prostatitis with
appropriate antimicrobial therapy
is often unrewarding
because of the poor diffusion
of most antimicrobials from the plasma
into the prostatic fluid.*

*Some success has recently been obtained
with the use of a combination of
trimethoprim and sulfamethoxazole.*

*The usual therapy is two weeks, but
longer periods of drug therapy may be
better and result in higher cure rates.*

*In patients not responding to the
combination of trimethoprim-
sulfamethoxazole . . .
either a course of minocycline . . . or
erythromycin-sodium bicarbonate
for two weeks may be used.*[1]

Possible Abscess

If the condition fails to respond to treatment it may be the indication of a _prostatic abscess_. In such a case, surgery is performed to drain the abscess.

---

[1] N. K. Bissada M.D., A. E. Finkbeiner, M.D., John F. Redman, M.D., Three Common Disorders of the Prostate (New York: Medical Times), February, 1977 (Vol. 105, No. 2), p. 54.

6

WHEN THE URINE STREAM DECREASES

PROSTATISM
(Benign Prostatic Hypertrophy)

The Enlarged Prostate

Upon examination of a male with this condition, the prostate is usually <u>enlarged</u> and firm in its consistency. The size of the prostate, however, (as determined by rectal digital examination) is a poor estimate of the degree of obstruction.

The doctor will usually watch a patient urinate *(void)* to check the consistency of the stream that comes from the penis. A decrease in the force or size of the stream may indicate an enlarged prostate that is benign and noncancerous and noninfectious.

If such a condition is not taken care of, it can lead to kidney stones or stones in the bladder or ureter. It can also lead to inflammation of the bladder, nephritis, kidney failure and uremia.

Symptoms

The doctor will look for symptoms such as:

1. Pain in prostate area
2. Discomfort in sitting
3. Frequent urination particularly at night
4. A small or dribbling stream when urinating
5. Low back pain
6. Premature ejaculation
7. Unexplained times of impotence

Antihistamines and anticholinergic drugs (atropine, belladonna, scopolamine) should be avoided.[1]

A Common Problem

When the bladder loses its ability to empty itself of all its urine because of the enlarged prostate, *residual urine* remains. It is estimated that about 70% of all men have some prostatic enlargement after the age of 60. Only about one out of five men with prostatic enlargement will require surgical relief for their symptoms.

Catheter Used to Empty Bladder

The doctor may pass a slender rubber tube (called a *catheter*) through the urethra into the bladder after the patient has urinated as much as he can. If urine still remains in the bladder, it is evident to the doctor that there is some obstruction that is preventing complete emptying.

Benign Prostatic Hypertrophy (BPH) is treated by a variety of techniques including cryogenic probes and cauterization. However, surgery is the most frequent approach to the problem. Surgery is usually

---

[1]Sigmund S. Miller, Symptoms (New York: Avon Books) 1978, p. 428.

used in one out of five men with this disease.

3 Approaches

Conservative initial treatment includes:

1. Drinking of ample quantities of water to stimulate emptying of the bladder and to prevent stagnation of urine.

2. Antibiotic drugs to prevent kidney infection or cystitis.

3. Sedatives or relaxant drugs to aid in urination.

Doctors generally recommend that alcoholic beverages and highly seasoned foods be avoided. They also suggest you stay away from very cold climates.

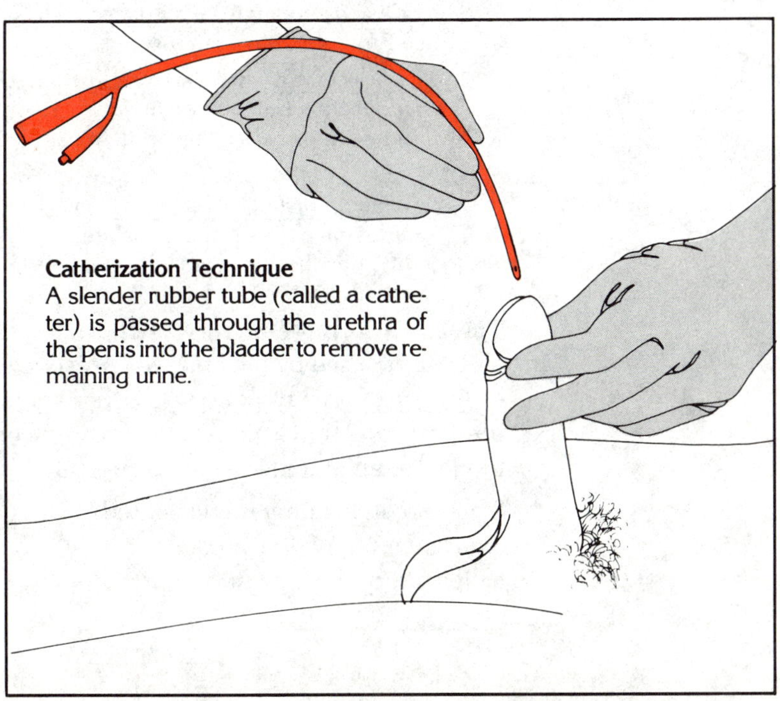

Catherization Technique
A slender rubber tube (called a catheter) is passed through the urethra of the penis into the bladder to remove remaining urine.

7

THE PROSTATE AND SURGERY

Determining Surgery

The doctor uses several guidelines to determine if surgery is required. They include:

1. <u>The amount of residual urine</u>
   The greater the amount of urine that remains behind after voiding, the greater is the need for surgical removal of the prostate.

2. <u>The severity of the symptoms</u>
   The more inconvenience that is produced by frequency of urination both by day and by night, the greater is the need for corrective surgery.

3. <u>The presence of associated conditions</u>
   Bladder infection, stones or a diverticulum will increase the need for surgery.

4. <u>Repeated episodes of hemorrhage</u>
   Hemorrhage from the prostate will point up the need for its surgical removal.[1]

The usual form of surgery to alleviate the blockage caused by the enlarged prostate is a <u>transurethral resection</u> (TUR). Transurethral resection is performed for small or moderate enlargements of the prostate.

<u>Open prostatectomy</u> is considered for large enlargements of the prostate. This is also called *suprapubic prostatectomy*.

---

[1]Robert E. Rothenberg, M.D., <u>The Complete Surgical Guide</u> (New York: Weathervane Books) 1974, p. 700.

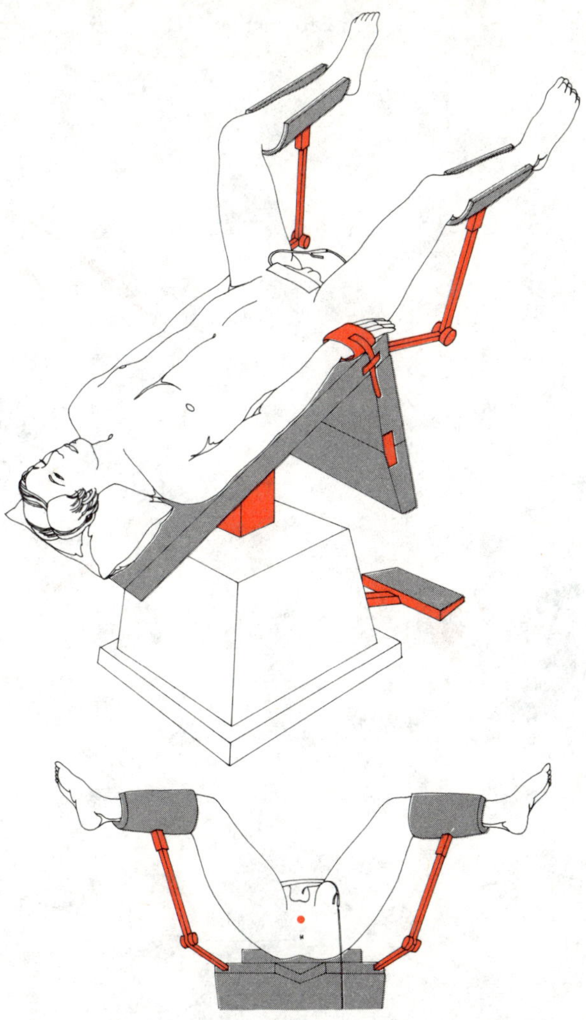

Illustration shows position of patient for <u>Perineal Prostatectomy</u>. <u>Top</u> picture indicates slant of operating table for this surgery. Note that penis is taped down during surgery.

<u>Bottom</u> picture shows position as viewed by surgeon. The incision site (red dot) is between the testicles and the anus.

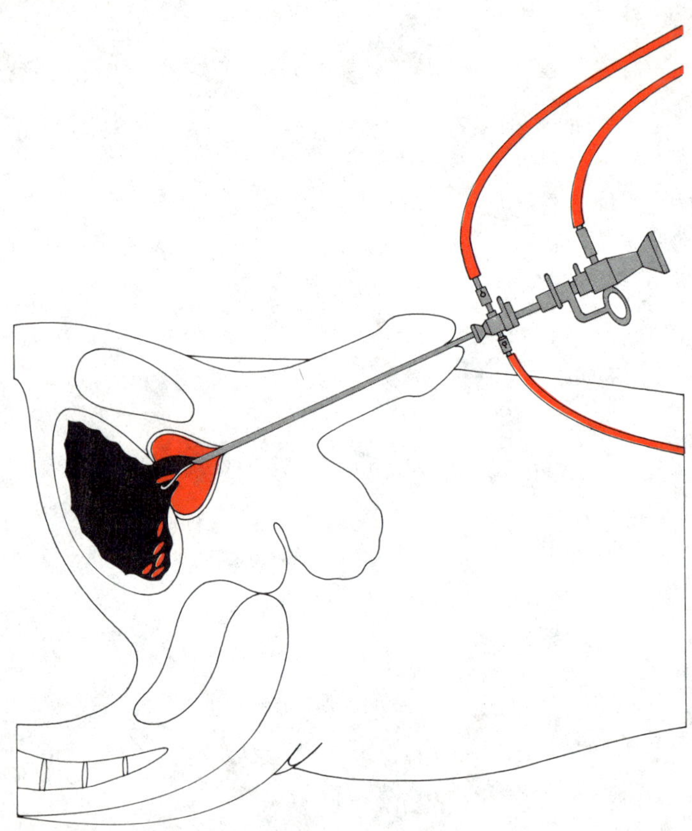

No incision is made in <u>Transurethral Resection</u>. A slender instrument is inserted through the channel of the penis *(urethra)*. It has a wire loop at its end which is electrically charged. The wire loop cuts away overgrown prostate tissue. The electric charge controls any bleeding.

TRANSURETHRAL RESECTION (TUR)

**No
Incision
Is
Made**

In transurethral resection (also called *transurethral prostatectomy*) no incision is made. The obstructing portion of the prostate is cut away by an electrically charged wire loop. This instrument, similar to a cystoscope but with a wire loop at its end, is introduced into the bladder through the penis.

The surgeon uses the wire loop to cut away chips of the inner portion of the prostate until all overgrown tissue is removed. The electrically charged wire loop controls any bleeding of the prostate gland.

Generally, a catheter is left in the bladder for several days after the operation. This is done to drain the urine until the prostate has a chance to heal. The hospital stay is usually one week and the patient can go back to work in about 3 weeks. About 70% of all patients can be treated by the transurethral resection technique. About 30% will require surgical incision. Normal voiding (urination) usually begins after 4-6 days.

Suprapubic Prostatectomy

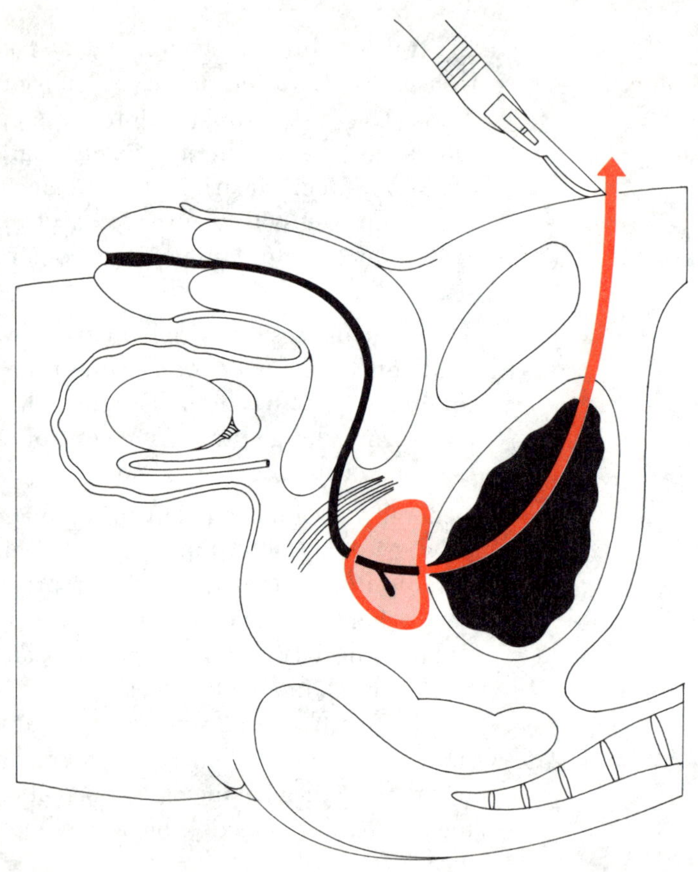

In <u>Suprapubic Prostatectomy</u>, the incision is made above the penis in the pubic area. The overgrown tissue of the prostate is removed <u>and a small incision is made into the bladder</u>. Catheters are left in place after the operation.

SUPRAPUBIC PROSTATECTOMY

Requires Incision In Abdomen

This form of surgery is performed if the prostate gland is very enlarged. The prostate is exposed through an incision in the lower abdomen. It is generally done as a one-step operation. The overgrown tissue is removed. The outer rim (the capsule) is left intact. Generally, two catheters are left in place after the operation. One is removed a few days later . . . the second in about one week.

The hospital stay is generally 12 days. One can go back to work in approximately 4 weeks.

Two-Stage Procedure

If there are complications, a two-stage procedure is followed.

> First, a *suprapubic cystostomy* in which the bladder is opened and drained through a small incision in the abdomen.

> Second, a few days or weeks later, the surgeon puts his finger in the opening in the bladder and removes the enlarged prostate.

Generally, both with the one-stage and two-stage operations, the tubes from the testicles *(vas deferens)* are cut and tied off. This is a vasectomy. It is done to prevent further infection called *epididymitis.*

A general or spinal anesthesia is used. Normal voiding (urination) usually begins after 10-14 days. Men do regain urinary control after a prostatectomy.

8

MEDICAL APPROACH TO PROSTATE CANCER

Cancer of the prostate seldom produces symptoms until it is well advanced. Generalized symptoms include: difficulty in starting urine stream, dribbling, unexplained cystitis and urine retention.

When the doctor checks out the prostate by way of a rectal examination he looks to see if there is a hard nodule in the prostate area. A <u>biopsy</u> confirms the presence of cancer. A *biopsy* is an excision of a small piece of tissue for microscopic examination.

About one half of the nodules examined are generally found to be malignant. Elevated serum acid phosphatase enzyme levels usually indicates prostatic cancer. Prostate cancer does not occur in eunuchs and is rare below the age of 30. A <u>eunuch</u> is a male who has had his testicles removed. It is estimated that in the United States some 5 million men are living with undetected cancer of the prostate.

There are four types of treatment for cancer of the prostate:

---

1. Radiation Therapy

This type of therapy is sometimes successful with locally contained cancer within the prostate when detected at an early stage.

2. Radical Prostatectomy

We have already described *suprapubic prostatectomy* on a previous page. This is one of <u>three</u> methods of <u>open surgical removal</u> of the prostate. The other two are:

Retropubic Prostatectomy
This is the most versatile procedure because the surgeon has direct eye vision of what he is doing. The prostate gland is removed directly through its coverings <u>without</u> making an incision in the bladder. This surgery has a shorter period of convalescence. The disadvantage is that the surgeon cannot treat any problems in the bladder that may be present. The incision for this surgery is made in the lower part of the abdomen.

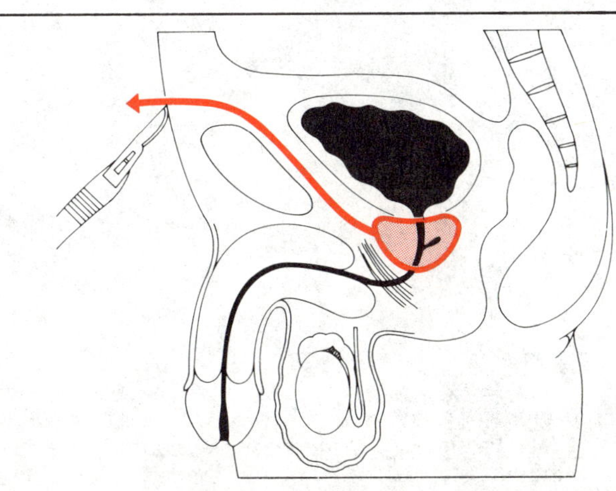

In <u>Retropubic Prostatectomy</u>, the incision is made above the penis in the pubic area. This surgery does <u>not</u> involve any incision into the bladder. This surgery has a shorter period of convalescence. Although the prostate is removed easier in this method, the surgeon cannot treat any problems in the bladder.

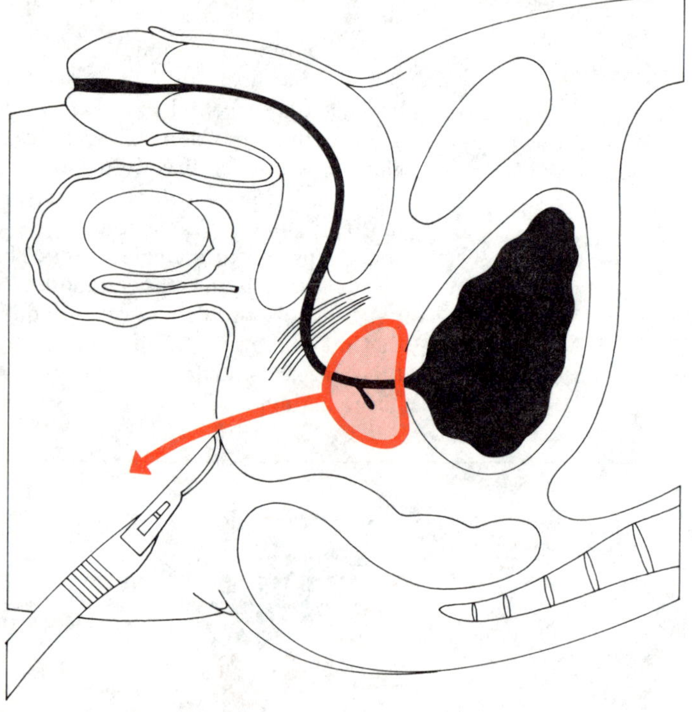

The <u>perineum</u> is the external area between the testicles and the anus. In <u>Perineal Prostatectomy</u>, the incision is made in this area for removal of the prostate. It is ideal surgery for the very old or for those with a large prostate as there is less incidence of shock.

**Chance
Of
Impotence**

Perineal Prostatectomy
This surgery is the same as Retropubic approach. The only difference is that the incision is made in the perineum. The perineum is the external area between the testicles and the anus. This method is preferred for radical cancer therapy. It has a low mortality rate and there is less incidence of shock. It is ideal for the very old and those with a large prostate.[1]

There is a greater chance of impotence with Perineal Prostatectomy because nerves and muscles that are involved in penile erection are severed in the course of this surgery.

---

3. Orchiectomy, Hormonal Therapy

**Testicles
Removed**

Sometimes when there is cancer of the prostate, the testicles are removed surgically. Removal has been found to slow down the growth and spread of the malignancy. Surgical removal of the testicles does not shorten life. It is still possible to have sexual intercourse after testicles have been removed. However, removal is usually only made in older men who are already impotent. The removal of the testicles stops the secretion of the male sex hormone. This surgery is called *orchiectomy*.

[1]Lillian S. Brunner, R.N., M.S.N., Doris S. Suddarth, R.N., M.S.N., Textbook of Medical-Surgical Nursing (Philadelphia: J. B. Lippincott Company) 1980, p. 1034.

Control Therapy

Hormonal therapy is a method of control rather than cure. It is sometimes called *Antiandrogen Therapy*. Diethylstilbestrol is the most widely used estrogen for this therapy. But it does have some annoying side effects. It causes *gynecomastia* (enlargement of breasts in the male). It can cause dizziness, lethargy, loss of appetite, diarrhea, constipation, excessive thirst, weight changes, impotence and migraine headaches. Its most dangerous side effect is the possibility of an em-bolism, the blocking of a blood vessel.

4. Chemotherapy and Hormonal Therapy

Combined Therapy

It is estimated that 70% of men with cancer of the prostate can receive some benefit from chemotherapy, according to those engaged in orthodox medicine. The usual chemotherapy drug used is *cyclo-phosphamide* which is Cytoxan. It is used with *doxorubicin* and *tamoxifen*. Side effects may include: abnormal decrease of white blood corpuscles, loss of appetite, nausea, vomiting, cystitis, sterility, loss of hair, hepatitis, along with cardiac problems.

POSSIBLE SIDE EFFECTS

Urine Leakage Disappears

After surgery, there is usually urinary incontinence. This is an inability to retain urine. This urine leakage may occur for several days but will disappear. After a prostatectomy, generally a three-way catheter is in place. After their removal the patient may have urinary frequency and burning upon urinating. This will disappear.

Ejaculation Force Lessened

In cancer of the prostate where a total prostatectomy is performed, impotence is almost always to be expected. If the patient does not want to give up sexual activity, a plastic insert may be used to make the penis rigid for sexual intercourse.

There is a theory that sexual activity may help to prevent prostate cancer. It is believed that sex hormones build up during abstinence and possibly reduce the prostate cells' immunity significantly.[1]

After any prostate surgery . . . if sexual intercourse is possible, the force of the ejaculation will be lessened.

---

[1]Medical Aspects of Human Sexuality/a monthly magazine published in New York.

All About PENILE IMPLANTS

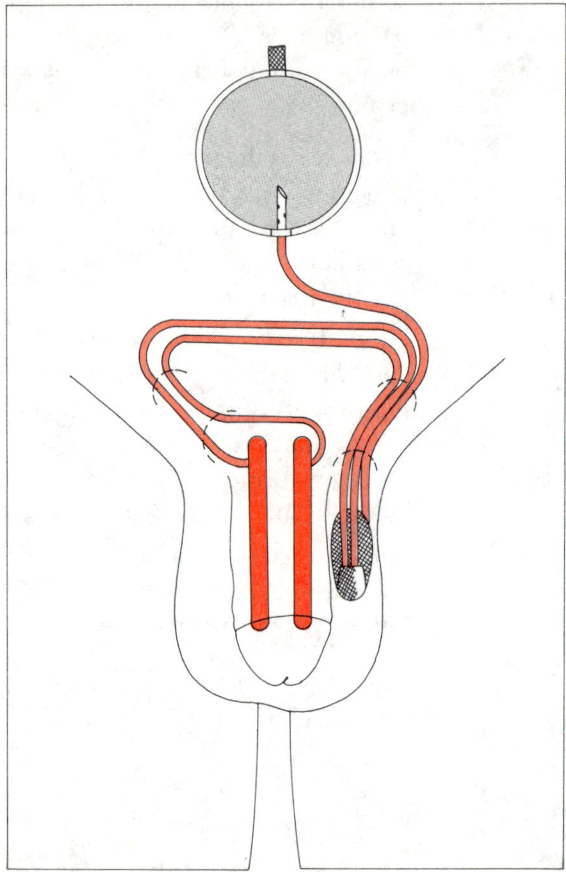

Illustrated is an <u>inflatable</u> <u>penile</u> <u>implant</u>. With this type of surgery, the individual can produce an erection only when it is desired. Two expansible, balloon-like cylinders made of silicone rubber are inserted into the erectile tissue on back of the penis. These cylinders connect to a reservoir **(see round circle)** on the abdominal wall near the bladder. Both male and female prefer this inflatable device rather than the <u>fixed</u> <u>rod</u> device.

2

All About PENILE IMPLANTS

A <u>penile implant</u> is sometimes referred to as a <u>penile prosthesis.</u> This is an artificial device that is placed in the penis to produce an erection.

This is implanted in the penis surgically and usually done under a local anesthetic. There are two types of implants: the fixed rod device and the inflatable device.

Fixed rod device

This is generally two semi-rigid silicone rods. The operation takes about one hour. The cost is some <u>$5000.</u> The disadvantage of this method is that one has a permanent semi-erection. This is sometimes called the <u>Small-Carrion penile prosthesis,</u> names after the originators. It can have both a psychological distress and cause some physical discomfort.

Inflatable device

The inflatable penile prosthesis produces an erection only when it is desired. The surgical insertion of this device is technically more difficult. The operation takes up to 90 minutes. Two expansible, balloon-like cylinders made of silicone rubber are inserted into the *corpora cavernosa* (two columns of erectile tissue on back of penis).

The cylinders are connected by tubing to a small spherical reservoir and to a tiny square pump. The reservoir is placed near the bladder <u>under</u> the muscles of the abdominal wall and filled with a saline solution. The pump is inserted into the scrotum. The cost for this operation is <u>over $6000.</u>

To bring an erection, the individual squeezes the pump several times. This forces fluid into the cylinders and swells the penis. After ejaculation, a release valve on the pump is opened. The salt solution blows back into the reservoir. The success rate is 99%. In studies taken, both the male and his female sexual partner prefer the inflatable device.

If a man is incapable of orgasm even with an erection, an implant will not help.

9

THE NUTRITIONAL APPROACH
TO
PROSTATE PROBLEMS

The Plague Of Modern Diets

Prostate problems are considered a disease that began in the 20th century. Could its emergence as a major disease be the result of modern diets deficient in vital nutrients due to over-processing of foods, the avoidance of fresh fruits and vegetables?

Among the nutrients processed out of our food that are vital to prostatic health are: magnesium, Vitamin F and zinc. The magnesium <u>deficiency</u> in the American diet is estimated at 200 milligrams a day.

Some prostate problems may be due to high-fat diets. That's the indication of studies by Carl P. Schaffner, Ph.D., professor of microbial chemistry at Rutgers University.

In another study made by the American Urological Association in 1976, high cholesterol levels appear to cause enlarged prostates.

Peter Hill, Ph.D., of the American Health Foundation in New York City conducted a test with a group of black South African volunteers.

**Rare
In
African**

He placed these black South African volunteers on a typical Western diet with lots of fats and meats. At the same time, a group of North American volunteers (black and white) were put on a low-fat diet. Dr. Hill tested for diet-induced hormonal changes that are associated with the development of prostatic cancer. (Prostatic cancer seems to be a hormonally associated disease.)

After three weeks, Dr. Hill found that the South Africans eating the Western diet were excreting notably more hormones, while the reverse occurred with the North Americans eating low-fat diet.[1]

This study indicates that a low-fat diet is one of the factors which can lower the risk of prostatic cancer.

Based on this study, some nutritionists suggest you substitute fruit and vegetable calories for animal calories.

INADEQUATE ZINC LEVELS

**Zinc
Essential
To
Prostate**

For 50 years it has been known that zinc is somehow essential to the health of the prostate gland. Prostatic fluid normally has an extraordinary concentration of zinc . . . about 7 milligrams per gram of fluid. It is also interesting to note that food processing eliminates much of zinc from the food

[1]Jonathan Uhlaner, Zinc, Fat and the Prostate (Emmaus, Pennsylvania: Prevention) April, 1980, p. 79.

The Airola Approach to Prostate Problems

Paavo Airola, a nutritionist, suggests several ways to alleviate prostate problems:

1. <u>Dietary</u>
   Emphasis on raw seeds and nuts especially pumpkin and squash seeds, sunflower seeds, almonds and sesame seeds. These foods are right in high quality proteins, unsaturated fatty acids and zinc. He also advocates raw vegetables and fruits, lecithin, brewer's yeast and Vitamin E. Avoid coffee, alcohol and all strong spices.

2. <u>Biological</u>
   Avoid sexual excitation without a natural conclusion in the form of ejaculation or orgasm. Prolonged engorgement, suppressed or incomplete ejaculation, withdrawal without orgasm may lead to functional and even structural damage of the prostate.

   <u>Prostate massage:</u> Lie flat on back, pull knees up as far as possible, then press the soles of both feet together. Holding soles pressed together, lower the legs as far as possible with a forceful movement. Repeat as many times as possible.

3. <u>Vitamins & Supplements (Daily)</u>
   Some of Dr. Airola's recommendations include:
   Pollen or pollen extract
      6 tables or 2 tablespoons of crude pollen
   F – essential fatty acids – 6 capsules
   E – 600 I.U.
   Chlorophyll perles
   Zinc supplement, organic – 30 milligrams
   C – 1000 mg. up to 5000 mg.
   Brewer's yeast – 2 tablespoons

   <u>Herbs</u>
   Juniper berry, ginseng, damiana, kelp, echinacea (for enlargement and weakness).[1]

Complete information on Dr. Airola's recommendations can be found in his book <u>How To Get Well</u>.

---

[1] Paavo Airola, Ph.D., N.D. <u>How To Get Well</u> (Phoenix, Arizona: Health Plus Publishers) 1976, pp. 143, 144.

we eat. In one study made at Mt. Sinai Medical Center in Chicago it revealed that more than one out of every three men did not have an adequate amount of zinc in the prostate.

Low Zinc Levels

A study in Chicago's Cook County Hospital showed that patients with chronic prostatitis or prostate cancer had low zinc levels.

When zinc therapy was administered to 200 patients having infectious prostatitis, 70% reported relief of their symptoms. Dr. Irving Bush of Chicago's Cook County Hospital gave each patient between 11 and 34 milligrams of zinc per day for up to 16 weeks.

BEE POLLENS REDUCES PROSTATE

Bee Pollen May Be Helpful

H. C. Mathews, at 78, had just had a medical examination and was told his prostate was fine considering his age. But Mathews was not reassured. He knew he was getting up every hour of every night to relieve the water pressure. He also had the memory of his brother's death 15 years prior. Cancer of the prostate was the cause.

He began to take bee pollen supplements. After six months of taking 8 pollen tablets daily, his prostate improved to the point where he could get 3-4 hours of uninterrupted sleep.

As the bee sucks nectar from the flower she also gathers pollen with the middle two of her six legs and packs it into the pollen baskets on her two hind-most legs.

When fully loaded, she flies home to the hive and packs the pollen into the honeycomb. It is this food that contains all the proteins, minerals and other nutrients necessary to transform the barely visible egg in six days to a larva the size of a full grown bee.

But now, some beekeepers use pollen traps attached to hive entrances. This forces the bee to crawl through a wire mesh that scrapes off the golden pellets from their hind legs. It is this that is compacted into tablets or granules for human use.[1]

Sex Hormones In Bee Pollen

A study published in a Yugoslav scientific journal, Experientia, reported that a tiny, yet potent amount of sex hormones are found in pollen. Pollen is rich in essential fatty acids, in minerals . . . of which it contains plentiful amounts of both magnesium and zinc (both beneficial to the prostate).

Gösta Jönsson, M.D., of the Urological Unit of the University of Lund, Sweden, observed that inflammatory changes of the prostate regressed with the use of bee pollen. Best results were obtained when 4 tablets were taken daily without interruption. No side effects were observed. Dr. Jönsson used a preparation known as Cer-

---

[1]H. C. Mathews, Tame That Prostate (Los Angeles: Let's Live) December, 1980, pp. 129, 131.

Another Remedy

nilton. Cernilton is basically pollen from timothy, maize and rye.[1]

Another study made in Japan at the Nagasaki University School of Medicine brought similar results.

A homeopathic home remedy for enlarged prostate includes a tincture which has Saw Palmetto, Chimaphila, Sulphur. About 15-20 drops are placed under the tongue three or four times daily.[2]

---

[1] Gösta Jönsson, M.D., Swedish Medical Journal (58:2487, 1961).

[2] Alan H. Nittler, M.D., Natra-Bio Homeopathic Home Remedies (Sumas, Washington: Botanical Laboratories, Inc.) 1997, p. 43.

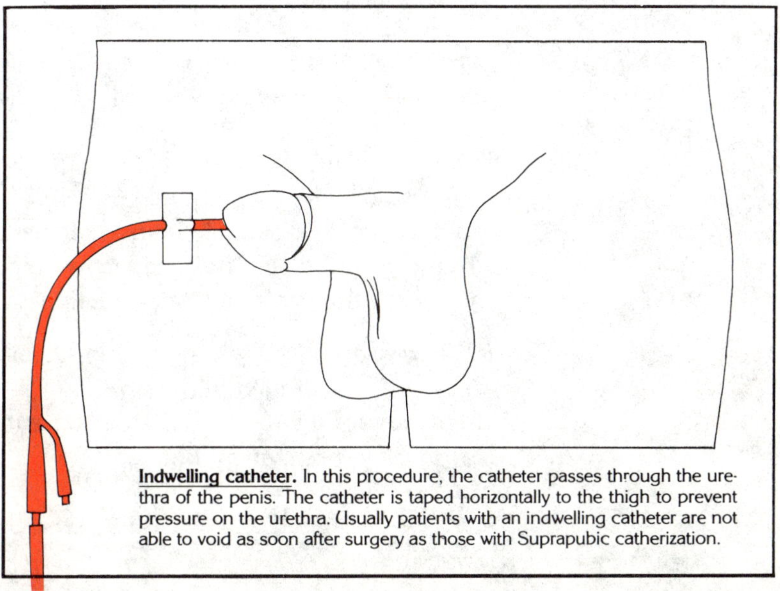

Indwelling catheter. In this procedure, the catheter passes through the urethra of the penis. The catheter is taped horizontally to the thigh to prevent pressure on the urethra. Usually patients with an indwelling catheter are not able to void as soon after surgery as those with Suprapubic catherization.

10

HERBS AND YOUR PROSTATE

HERBS EASE DISTRESS

**Three
Herbs
Therapeutic**

Herbs are sometimes recommended for prostate distress. Dr. George Zofchak is an herbalist, chiropractor and naturopath who specializes in herb therapy. He suggests:

> *The three major herbs
> indicated to ease prostate distress are
> buchu leaves
> uva-ursi
> saw palmetto.*
>
> *Buchu leaves are especially valued
> for soothing irritation to the bladder.*[1]

William R. Fair, M.D. working with researchers at the Washington University School of Medicine in St. Louis reported that <u>zinc</u> has antibacterial properties and may protect the prostate from infection.

**Zinc
Deficiency
Noted**

In this research the prostatic fluid was examined from 15 men with chronic prostatitis. They found an average zinc content of 50 <u>micrograms</u> per milliliter. But when

---

[1]Mark Bricklin, <u>The Practical Encyclopedia of Natural Healing</u> (Emmaus, Pennsylvania: Rodale Press) 1976, p. 219.

they examined 49 men who were free of prostatitis, they found an average zinc content almost nine times higher: 448 micrograms per milliliter.[1]

PUMPKIN SEEDS KILL PARASITES

Pumpkin Seeds Suggested

LaDean Griffin believes, if no cancer is evident, that swelling of the prostate is often pockets of worms in the lower bowel, causing both irritation and eventual swelling. Mrs. Griffin has been a nutritionist and herbalist for over 25 years. She suggests the method to kill the parasites or worms is pumpkin seed. She believes all men over 40 would do well to eat a handful of pumpkin seed every day as a preventive food.

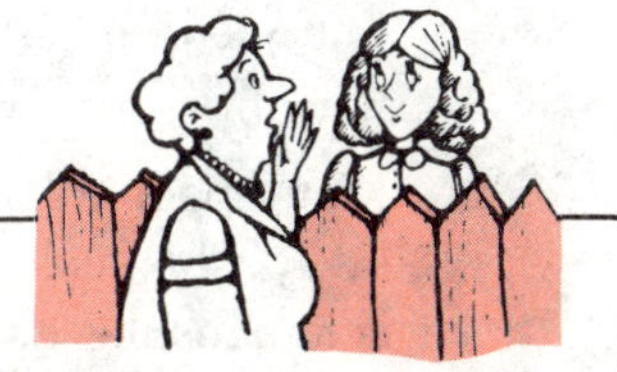

AUNT EFFIE . . .
Did Angus have a Prostate problem?

You could always tell the time of night. Angus would get up 3 or 4 times a night. Finally, I put him wise. Take some zinc tablets and pumpkin seed oil every day, I told him. He finally minded me and now he can make it through the night. Changed his eating habits, too. Eats a fresh pear daily!

---

[1]Medical World News, February 7, 1977.

HERBALIST SUGGESTS GINSENG

**Ginseng
A
Hormonal Herb**

Male hormone herbs to aid the prostate, according to LaDean Griffin are sarsaparilla and ginseng. She suggests:

> *The use of Ginseng as a male hormone*
> *acts in a similar way*
> *to the drug testosterone*
> *which merely gives strength and vigor*
> *to the male; and Ginseng*
> *does not have the side effects*
> *of testosterone.*
>
> *It would be well for all men over 40*
> *to learn the uses of Ginseng.*
> *In the herb world,*
> *it is a must to be used along*
> *with any cancer formulas*
> *where prostate cancer is present.*[1]

Hormonal herbs, states LaDean Griffin, do not have the side effects that are found in hormone drugs.

Many people have found relief from prostate problems by taking 3 unsaturated fatty acid capsules daily (Vitamin F). Others, eat a handful of pumpkin seeds daily.

---

[1]LaDean Griffin, Prostate Problems and The Male Hormone (Salt Lake City, Utah: The Herbalist) 1976, Vol. 1, No. 9, pp. 343, 344.

11

ENEMAS AND THE PROSTATE

3 ENEMIES OF HEALTHY PROSTATE

Some Causes of the Problem

Many of those engaged in natural healing techniques believe that prostate problems stem from a combination of causes.

1. <u>Overeating</u>
   As we get older there is a tendency to eat as much or more as when we were young. This places a strain on the body since we do not work off this excess food. The prostate can eventually suffer.

2. <u>Constipation</u>
   This causes congestion in the tissues of the rectum, spreading to the prostate. The laxative habit compounds the insults to this sensitive area.

3. <u>Sedentary occupation</u>
   It has been said that "... *footprints in the sands of time are not made sitting down...*." Sitting or standing in one position for a long period of time has a direct effect on the circulatory system which eventually includes the prostate.

As one gets older, if he allows himself to have a sagging abdomen, prostate problems can develop. A heavy, overloaded abdomen places downward pressure on the bladder and can cause urine retention.

The MORRISON Approach To PROSTATE PROBLEMS

Marsh Morrison is widely regarded as the *"Dean"* of American chiropractors. He has practiced for over 40 years. He is now retired but is often called upon for consultation by European royalty and other prominent people. He is the author of 23 books on natural healing.

For prostatitis . . . inflammation of the prostate gland . . . Dr. Morrison has several suggestions. He has what he terms Four Steps To Health to open up the nerve supply to the ailing prostate.

    1. Cold Water Soak

Soak buttocks in a small shallow basin filled with cold water. Keep water cold by adding ice cubes. Dr. Morrison states that this shrinks the swollen gland, pulling it away from the urethra. This should make it easier for you to urinate.

    2. Elbows and Knees Exercise Position

This exercise is designed to strengthen a particular group of muscles which pulls the inside of the prostate away from the urethra.

As reported in The Healthview Newsletter

Get on your elbows and knees . . . close to the edge of the bed so that your head overhangs the edge and rests downward.

In this position, blow out your breath and suck the rectum toward the belly-button. Hold as long as you can . . . then release the tension and inhale a new breath. Then repeat the process 6 or 7 times.[1]

---

[1]Sam Biser, The Healthview Newsletter (Box 6670, Charlottesville, Virginia) 1978, No. 16, p. 6. Copies of the complete interview may be secured by sending $2 direct to The Healthview Newsletter.

3. The Cleansing Process

To cleanse the prostate gland of toxic and irritating debris, Dr. Morrison suggests that the individual eats nothing but fruits for an entire week. He states that any fruit can be eaten ... but two fruits that are especially beneficial are:

> Bartlett pears
> Watermelon

In eating watermelon he recommends that the fruit be cut into small cubes ... bite size. Eat one of these cubes every 5-10 minutes all day. Don't drink or eat anything else that day. This procedure will cause you to urinate quite frequently eliminating wastes from your body.

After this one day watermelon cleansing, Dr. Morrison suggests the individual refrains from drinking any liquids or juicy fruits and vegetables for several days. Instead eat other nutritional foods. Such a procedure gives your bladder and prostate a rest.

4. Rectal Massage

He next suggests rectal dilation. This is intended to release muscle tension in the groin area. It is his theory that this allows fresh blood to enter the prostate and heal it. He also recommends it for releasing nervous tension.

For a rectal massage he suggests one obtains a rectal dilator and a tube of K-Y jelly or wheat germ oil. Rectal dilators come in several sizes from small to large. Start with the small dilator. Lubricate it. Insert it in your rectum while lying on your left side (or on your hands and knees). He suggests that the dilator will probably go in 3 to 4 inches. Once inserted, the circular muscles (*anal sphincters*) will grip the rectal dilator holding it in place.

Maintain this position for about 15 minutes. This exercise may be done several times a week or every day, if needed. He recommends it best be done just before bedtime.

Dr. Morrison suggests this exercise activates the nerve center called the *Impar Ganglion* which, in turn, stimulates the heart, thyroid, pituitary, genitals and appendix.

For diet, Dr. Morrison suggests an individual eats more fresh raw greens. He suggests limiting protein to 4 ounces of seeds or nuts ... or 8 ounces or less of steak, chicken, fish, turkey or cottage cheese.

He believes that halibut, mackerel and red snapper fish supply a lot of natural iodine which improves the functioning of the sexual organs.

He also recommends that one refrains from sex while the prostate is healing. The healing process using natural non-surgical methods takes about 6 to 8 weeks, according to Dr. Morrison.

Dr. Morrison, in an interview with the Editor of The Healthview Newsletter, remarked:

> *... the nerves that serve the prostate gland*
> *leave the spinal column*
> *at the lower vertebrae in your back.*
>
> *I've never seen even a single case*
> *of prostatitis in which*
> *one or more nerves were not blocked*
> *or pinched*
> *somewhere along their route to the prostate—*
> *cutting off the free flow of nerve power to it.*
>
> *... every prostate patient I've ever had*
> *did respond positively*
> *once I showed him how to reestablish*
> *the flow of healing life forces*
> *back to the organ.*[1]

Dr. Morrison believes that these natural healing forces can work even if a man has cancer of the prostate.

---

[1] Ibid., Number 15, p. 3.

Besides the water diet as described in the Morrison approach to prostate problems . . . some suggest an <u>enema</u> program. This cleansing of the colon is thought to be beneficial.

THE COLD WATER ENEMA

**Taken
At Night**

One variation of the enema program is what is called the <u>Cold Water Enema.</u>

A pint of <u>cold</u> (not lukewarm) water is injected into the lower bowel every evening upon retiring. It is injected in slowly and should be retained for up to about 30 minutes. This is done every night for one week; then every other night for another week; and then every weekend for a month.

**Helps
Hemorrhoids**

This cold water enema program is believed by some nutritionists to have a beneficial effect on the prostate. It is also believed to be of great value in helping to clear up hemorrhoids and improving the general tone of the rectal tissues.

ALL ABOUT ENEMAS

In Louis XIV's day, enemas were a fad. Many women in royalty had enemas three times a day. In fact the King himself had 107 assorted doctors and in one year they administered to the King 215 enemas.[1]

Enema means *"to throw in"* and medically they are usually given by injecting a liquid solution into the rectum and colon to empty the lower intestine or to introduce food or medicine for therapeutic purposes. A regular enema reaches only about 5 or 6 inches of the colon.

A **high enema** is designed to reach the colon. Thus a long rubber 30 inch tube is extended into the rectum to carry the cleansing liquid as far up as possible in the colon.

Basically there are **four** types of enemas:

1. Barium enema
   Administration of barium sulfate in solution as a diagnostic aid in X-ray examination of the colon.
2. Carminative enema
   One given to relieve distention caused by flatus (gas) and to stimulate peristalsis.
3. Cleansing enema
   One to empty the lower intestine or the colon. Often a coffee enema is used for this process.
4. Retention enema
   A coffee enema is considered a retention enema in that the liquid is retained in the colon for a period of time. Retention enemas are used also to soothe or lubricate the rectal mucous membrane, to apply absorbable medication or to soften feces.

How To Take An Enema

To take an enema, you must have an enema can or bag with a rubber hose and a nozzle; it can be obtained at any drug store.

Fill the enema bag with lukewarm water, about 99 degrees F. Add a few drops of fresh lemon juice, or a cup of camomile tea (can be bought at health food stores); however, the enema can be taken with plain water. For a do-it-yourself enema, 1 pint to 1 quart water is sufficient.

---

[1]Marian T. Troy, Better Bowel Health (New York: Pyramid Books), 1974, p.180.

The best position for taking an enema is on your knees, head down to the floor, with enema bag hanging 12 to 18 inches above the anus, to get sufficient pressure in the flow of water. The flow can be regulated by squeezing the tube with the fingers; some enema bags have a special clamp to regulate the flow.

Before inserting the nozzle into the anus, make sure there is no air left in the tube; let water run for a moment. Use some vaseline, oil or other lubricant on the nozzle to make insertion easier. If you feel discomfort or pain when water is running in, stop the flow for a while and take a few deep breaths; then continue again until the bag is empty.

If you can retain the water for a while and do not feel forced to empty the bowels at once, you may lie on a bed or soft rugs for a few minutes and let the water do its dissolving and washing work before letting it out. First lie on the back for a minute, then on the right side, then on the stomach, and then on the left side. While you are doing this, gently massage your stomach with your hands. Then go to the toilet and let the water out. Stay long enough to make sure the bowels are empty.

For a small child or a baby, a small all-rubber-bulb ear syringe can be used. The tip of the bulb should be lubricated with petroleum jelly. Do not use soapy water. For an infant, use up to 4 ounces of luke warm plain water. For a 1-year-old, up to 8 ounces of water. For a 5-year-old, up to one pint. Gently insert the lubricated syringe tip into the anus. The slower you inject the solution, the more effective the enema will be. Hold the child's buttocks together to prevent a premature evacuation.

Enemas are preferred over laxatives because there are fewer dangers of sensitivity, allergies and interference with normal bowel functions. Diabetics do not have to worry about sugar nor the heart patient about sodium (as they would if they took a laxative) because an enema only reaches the colon.

An enema has the advantage in that it acts quickly . . . within a few minutes. Enemas, too, have a soothing effect and are safer to use in cases of constipation than laxatives.

WHEN SEXUAL URGE DIMINISHES

Often in the early stages of prostate problems one may complain of a dull, aching pain in the nape of the neck . . . right up close to the skull and usually more to the left side. There may be a feeling of depression and a loss of sex drive. This may be mistaken as the "*male climacteric*" or male "*change of life*" when in reality it is a prostate problem.

When Sexual Desires Wane

The lessening of sexual desires, the inability to maintain an erection or properly perform the sex act can all be indications of a pesky prostate. The appearance of a thin, mucous-like, oily substance trickling from your penis, where there is no sexual stimulation, may indicate a prostate problem.

When sexually excited, the preliminary fluid that trickles down comes from the Cowpers glands into the urethra neutralizes any acidity left there by urine. An abnormal discharge is called *prostatorrhea*.

Many people with prostate problems have been found to be heavy users of salt or monosodium glutamate, which is a form of salt.

Lack Of Essential Oils

The late John H. Tobe suggested in his book, <u>Your Prostate</u> that the most important cause of prostate problems is a lack of natural essential oils in the body. Most of the oils we take into our body today are highly refined or chemically treated, heated or synthesized. He suggests:

> *Each ejaculation costs*
>   *a man something . . .*
> *he is giving something of his body*
> *and something of himself.*
>
> *It is also recognized that the semen*
> *is an oily substance.*
>
> *Remember, nature must continually*
> *replenish this supply of oily*
> *seminal fluid.*[1]

Seeds Suggested

To restore natural essential oils, John Tobe recommends

> Pumpkin seeds
> Squash seeds
> Sunflower seeds
> Sesame seeds
> Flax seeds

Tobe mixed flax, sesame and honey in equal parts and stirred them up as an aid.

Tobe believed that sexual intercourse plays a vital part in maintaining a healthy prostate. He wrote:

> *It is my opinion that*
> *from youth to middle age*
> *a man in good health*
> *should require sexual indulgence*
> *from 3 to 7 times a week.*[2]

---

[1] John H. Tobe, <u>Your Prostate, Treatment and Prevention</u> (St. Catharines, Ontario, Canada: Provoker Press) 1968, p. 209.

[2] Ibid., p. 124

He maintained that a healthy man in his 60's or 70's should be able to achieve the same performance.

SEX FOR HEALTHY PROSTATE

Surgical Aftereffects

Tobe suggests that some unhappy results can occur after a prostatectomy operation in which the prostate is removed.

First, the man most likely will be made impotent.

Second, if the wife is an introvert, having lived completely for her husband . . . when her husband shows no further interest in her sexually . . . she may deteriorate mentally.

ADVICE FOR WIVES

Tobe believed that proper sexual relations encourage a healthy prostate and writes this advice to wives:

> Women,
>   if you want a sexually virile husband
>   if you want a loving mate,
>   if you want a man
>   who will have his prostate
>   and thus be able to enjoy sex
>   with you for many long years,
>   provide him with
>   sexual intercourse
>   whenever he desires it . . .
>
> I think it is cheap
> health and life insurance.[1]

[1]Ibid., p. 205.

Avoid Congestion

Tobe saw the prostate gland as one that functioned healthfully as it kept flowing. A husband who needs sexual intercourse 4 or 5 times a week . . . and who is restricted by a wife who only provides it once or twice a week . . . (by her refusals) backs up her husband's prostate fluid. Congestion develops and finally prostate problems ending in possible surgical removal of the prostate. That's how Tobe and other nutritionists view the situation.

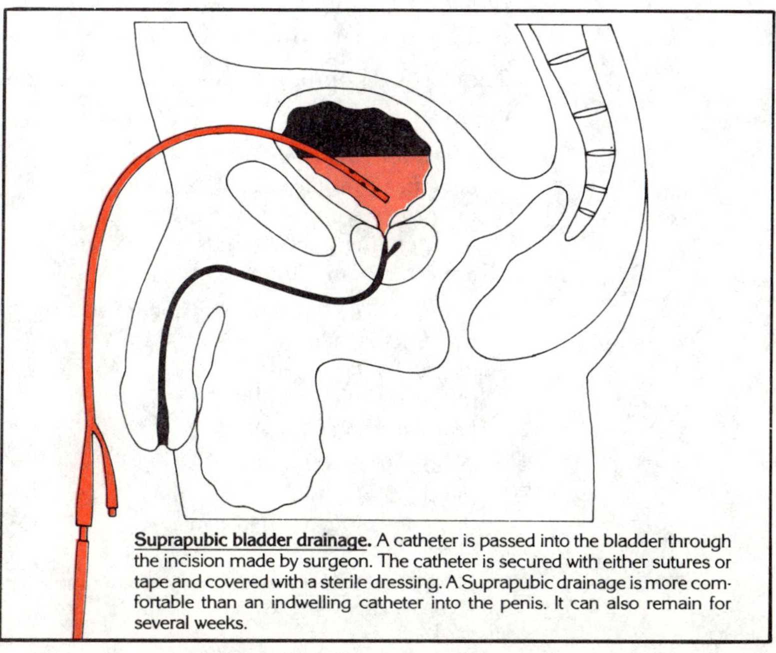

Suprapubic bladder drainage. A catheter is passed into the bladder through the incision made by surgeon. The catheter is secured with either sutures or tape and covered with a sterile dressing. A Suprapubic drainage is more comfortable than an indwelling catheter into the penis. It can also remain for several weeks.

13

PROSTATE AND SEXUAL INTERCOURSE

Prolonged
Sex

COITUS PROLONGATUS

John Tobe has coined a phrase which is not found in medical textbooks. He calls it *Coitus Prolongatus*. He defines this by comparing it to an automobile. You start the car and eventually reach 60 m.p.h. then slow down your engine to almost a standstill . . . then accelerate to full speed again. This repeated on and off procedure, Tobe states, will soon wear down your car engine.

Then Tobe compares this to sexual intercourse:

> *All conditions leading to the sex act*
> *have been fulfilled . . . it is in motion . . .*
> *the prostate and*
> *its attending ducts, glands and organs*
> *are functioning in unison.*
>
> *Then, just as the climax is about reached*
> *and finis is to be written to the act*
> *(as nature intended)*
> *the process is abruptly*
> *brought to a standstill.*
>
> *Then in a few minutes*
> *the process is repeated . . . and*
> *this goes on again and again.*[1]

---

[1] John H. Tobe, Your Prostate, Treatment and Prevention (St. Catharines, Ontario, Canada: Provoker Press) 1968, p. 209.

This prolonged action, Tobe suggests, is not normal and repeated swelling and diminishing eventually brings hypertropy (enlargement) of the prostate.[1]

COITUS INTERRUPTUS

Withdrawal Damaging

Coitus Interruptus is the withdrawal of the penis from the vagina before the seminal emission occurs. This form of sexual intercourse is practiced sometimes in order to avoid pregnancy. The ejaculation is spilled outside the vagina.

In the Old Testament of the Bible in the book of Genesis 38:1:11, Onan was commanded by his father to marry his brother's wife, Tamar. Onan's brother was killed by the Lord and so it was Onan's responsibility to take over the duty as husband to Tamar.

In Levitical law, any sons from Tamar would then be Onan's brother's heirs. Onan was not willing to have a child who would not be counted as his own. So although he married Tamar . . . whenever he went in to sleep with her, he spilled the sperm on the bed to prevent her from having a baby. Be-

[1]For complete information on sexual problems, you may want to secure The Medical Approach versus The Nutritional Approach To Impotence and Frigidity by Salem Kirban. Send a total of $6 ($1 is for postage) to: Salem Kirban, Inc., Kent Road, Huntingdon Valley, Pennsylvania 19006.

cause Onan did not fulfill his responsibility, the Lord also killed him.

<u>Coitus Interruptus</u> builds to a climax that is not completely fulfilled. Continued practice of this nature, some believe, may add repeated insults to the prostate. Tobe likens the prostate as a shock absorber that through misuse, finally enlarges.

COITUS RESERVATUS

**Suppression
Unnatural**

<u>*Coitus Reservatus*</u> is sexual intercourse with intentional suppression of ejaculation.

There was a group called the Oneida Community which believed that the useless expenditure of semen continually is not natural. They practiced sexual intercourse without the male releasing his sperm. In some Yoga circles this also is practiced. They claim that sexual communion can be indulged in for 8-10 hours without losing a drop of semen. This act is called <u>*carrhiza*</u>.

There are some who believe that this other than normal procedure can eventually cause the prostate to enlarge.

A similar suppression of ejaculation is called <u>*Coitus Soxonius*</u>. In this procedure, manual pressure is placed on the urethra at the underside of the penis to block the emission of semen at the time of ejaculation.

Such interruptions of the sexual procedure may eventually cause an enlarged prostate and other problems.

Forcing Orgasm Harmful

Many in the medical profession also believe that masturbation and the forcing of an orgasm is one of the leading causes of prostate problems.

The MINERAL Approach To Illness
An Interview with Paul Eck

Dr. Paul Eck has a degree in the field of <u>naprapathy.</u> Naprapathy is a system of therapy which attributes all disease to disorders of the nervous system, ligaments and connective tissue.

He is director of Analytical Research Laboratories in Phoenix, Arizona which specializes in interpreting hair tests. Paul Eck prepares vitamin and mineral programs for many medical doctors and other health practitioners.

Dr. Eck has very definite views on how to correct basic illnesses. They differ quite dramatically from the standard medical approach to disease. In fact, they differ also from many of the usual nutritional approaches to disease, as well!

Dr. Eck believes that much of what is going on today in the field of nutrition is guesswork. Too many people are spending anywhere from $5000 to $15,000 to correct health deficiences and are no better off physically. The problem, as Eck sees it, is that it is not the products they are taking that are wrong . . . but that the necessary knowledge and application to <u>utilize</u> these various nutrients is missing!

In an interview with Sam and Loren Biser of <u>The Healthview Newsletter</u>, Eck commented:

> *It's not the amount of vitamins that you take nor is it the amount of minerals you are taking or anything else . . . the products or the money that you are spending . . . I think a lot of this is pure waste because if it is not being applied in a scientific way there's no way that it's ever going to work!*[1]

---

[1]Paul Eck, <u>Your Minerals and Your Health</u> (To secure this one hour cassette, send $10 direct to Healthview Newsletter, Box 6670, Charlottesville, Virginia 22906)

Other cassettes by Dr. Paul Eck on various metabolic dysfunctions and philosophy of health are available from Analytical Research Laboratories, Inc., 2338 West Royal Palm Road, Suite F, Phoenix, Arizona 85021.

The MINERAL Approach To Illness
An Interview with Paul Eck

When Paul Eck first became interested in hair analysis he discovered he had a low zinc level of 9 (the normal zinc level is 20). He also had hypoglycemia, he was nervous and had a tendency towards diabetes. He also knew his anxiety levels were high.

To try and correct his low zinc level he began taking 3 zinc tablets a day. He was surprised to find that he did not get better. In fact, he became worse and experienced extreme fatigue. He decided to go off the zinc and his energy level began to come back to what it was before.

Simply adding zinc to your system can cause other problems. Too much zinc has a tendency to make your copper level low. The normal level for copper in the human body, according to Eck, is 2.5mg./% He states that anyone with a copper level of 1.0 is in a potential cancerous state.

Low copper levels symptoms may show up as: fatigue, anemia, joint pain and depression. Eck believes this can lead to a cancerous condition because:

> ... *the copper inside the cell regulates the respiratory oxidation mechanism which prevents you from getting cancer.*[1]

Paul Eck also says that if one has a high copper level ... and takes a multiple vitamin/mineral tablet or supplement that has copper in it, their physical problem will become worse. The additional copper, adding to their already high level, will accentuate their illness and the other vitamins and minerals in the daily supplement will be of no value. The indiscriminate taking of vitamins and minerals can be a hit and miss type of therapy. It can be a total waste of money, according to Eck. He believes that up to 90% of the people taking multiple vitamin supplements are damaging their health.

Eck states that copper is the most dangerous of all the required minerals, if you are not aware of what your body requires. Simply to take copper supplements on a guess-basis can be hazardous to your health.

---

[1]Ibid.

The MINERAL Approach To Illness
An Interview with Paul Eck

Paul Eck also believes that excessive Vitamin C taken over a considerable length of time and in certain "biological types" can cause cancer. He suggests that soils that are high in calcium and magnesium protect against cancer. Any mineral, therefore, that can lower these two minerals (calcium and magnesium) or copper can cause a cancerous condition.

In a recorded interview for <u>The Healthview Newsletter,</u> Eck stated:

> *There is no question that a person can take Vitamin C in some cancer cases and derive results.*
>
> *But, just as zinc lowers copper, which is perhaps the most protective mineral against cancer ... Vitamin C also has a copper lowering effect, and over the years, can cause cancer.*[1]

Dr. Paul Eck does not believe it is necessary in the majority of cases to give large doses of Vitamin C. He says that copper makes up a part of an enzyme called <u>ascorbic acid oxidase.</u> An <u>oxidase</u> is a catalyst. It is the copper in this formula that activates the enzyme. If this ascorbic acid oxidase enzyme is missing, Eck believes then that Vitamin C cannot be oxidized to adequate amounts in the body. Therefore, Eck concludes, if this optimal oxidation is not taking place, large amounts of Vitamin C are not only useless but can initiate various disease proccesses.

If your body is not functioning properly, the vitamins will not excrete the excess minerals you may be taking in your daily supplements. Instead they accumulate in the body. If your body is deficient in Vitamin B[6], as an example, you will have a tendency to accumulate copper in the body. This can result in a <u>toxic</u> level of <u>copper</u> in your system.

Dr. Eck does not encourage the taking of multiple vitamins and minerals. He feels this indiscrimate use is detrimental to one's health ... since every individual is biochemically different.

---

[1]Ibid.

4
The MINERAL Approach To Illness
An Interview with Paul Eck

Paul Eck is a firm believer in using hair analysis tests.

> *A hair analysis test is the only method developed that has any validity at all as far as measuring what actually is occurring in the tissues of the body.*
>
> *It has the benefit of being able to give you a metabolic pattern of every metabolic activity that is occurring in your body over a period of time.*[1]

Dr. Eck believes that blood tests, in this context, are frequently invalid because they give you an up-to-the-minute readout. It is not a true reflection of what is happening in the tissues over a period of time. A person taking a high amount of Vitamin C could be releasing from his system large amounts of cholesterol. If a blood test were taken at that time it would show a high cholesterol level. However, what the physician does not realize is that it is not a build-up of cholesterol but, quite the opposite, a beneficial flushing of cholesterol out of the body.

Too many people, Dr. Eck suggests, take maganese when they have a manganese deficiency . . . they take iron when they have an iron deficiency, etc. **This is wrong.** To give iron to raise iron is to lower iron!

Dr. Louis Kervan, in his book, Biological Transmutations makes the following observations:

> For IRON deficiency . . . give Manganese.
> For MANGANESE deficiency . . . give Copper.
> For MAGNESIUM deficiency . . . give Zinc.
> For ZINC deficiency . . . give Magnesium.

Prostate Problems

Prostate problems are associated with one or more mineral ratio imbalances. The most prominent imbalance involves disturbed sodium/magnesium ratio.

The optimal ratio is **4.16** parts of sodium to **one** part of magnesium. When the sodium/magnesium ratio becomes greater than **16/1** an inflammatory process is initiated which can involve the prostate gland. This is particularly so if zinc levels are also low.

---

[1]Ibid.

The MINERAL Approach To Illness
An Interview with Paul Eck

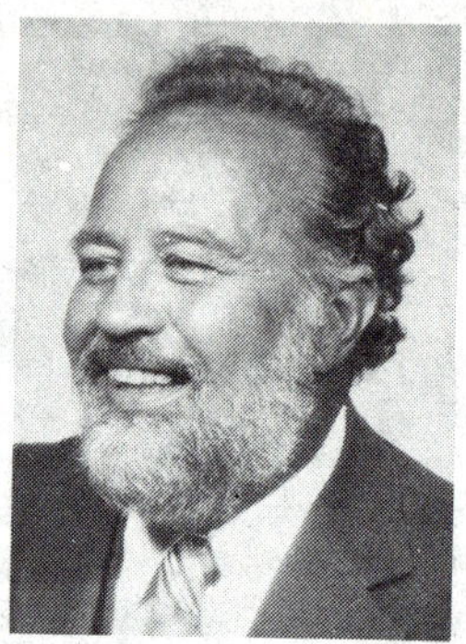

When you go on a correct vitamin/ mineral supplementation, the excess minerals and toxic minerals (such as cadmium, lead, aluminum) will start to unload and flush out of your system. This unloading will cause headaches and numerous other symptoms which will vary with the toxic metal or combination of toxic metals being eliminated, and in some cases make you feel worse. This is a natural occurrence as your body gets rid of these unwanted elements to get you on the road to full recovery.

Dr. Eck believes that mineral imbalances should be corrected mainly by using <u>small</u> potency vitamins and minerals. He says it just takes a very small amount of a mineral to initiate a major physiological process in the body. Any amount over that, he states, will cause exactly the opposite reaction.

Paul Eck believes that mineral therapy is also indirectly hormone therapy. Through the results found in hair analysis he has been able to see people go off hormone therapy, estrogen, even off of thyroxin. He has used manganese and copper to improve their thyroid function where indicated.

Paul Eck is very familiar with Diabetes. His grandmother, his mother was diabetic. He and his brother were pre-diabetic. Dr. Eck states he can determine from a hair analysis, years in advance, whether a person will become a diabetic.

Paul Eck says that 90% of the people who have diabetes have more than enough insulin circulating in their blood. When you have a low calcium to magnesium ratio (such as 3.3 to 1) you have an individual that has diabetes. And if the ratio is high, such as <u>10</u> parts calcium to <u>1</u> part magnesium . . . you are in the diabetic area.[1]

Eck states:

> *One problem in about 10% of the diabetics is the lack of calcium in the pancreas. This condition results in an inability of the Islets of Langerhans to secrete insulin . . .*

---

[1]The calcium to magnesium <u>ratio</u> normally is 6.7 to 1. This means for every 1 part of magnesium in your system, you should have 6.7 parts of calcium.

because when the calcium drops below a certain level you can't even initiate the secretion of the insulin that is manufactured and is being stored in pancreatic Islets of Langerhans tissue.

So what you have to do is, by one means or another, raise the calcium level back up to a close to normal ratio between the magnesium and then you automatically get a secretion of insulin.

This occurs in your insulin-deficiency diabetics ... which only accounts for about 10 or 12% of the cases.

Dr. Eck states that the rest of the problem in diabetes lies either in the <u>transport of the insulin to the cell itself</u> or, when it gets to the cell, there is a <u>lack of a receptor</u> at the cell site on the cell membrane. Those receptors are all <u>minerals!</u> Therefore, Dr. Eck concludes:

If the proper mineral is not available in the body for transport of the insulin to the cell ... it doesn't get there in the first place.

Secondly, even when it gets there, if some receptor is not present, and there are multiple receptors on the cell membrane ... then, of course, the insulin can't even enter the cell and do what it is supposed to do!

We have had such great reports especially in diabetes.

You know the old saying that says "Once you've been on insulin, you're going to stay on it the rest of your life ..." that's the same statement they use for hypothyroidism. They say: "Once you're on thyroid, you're going to be on it forever. Make up your mind to it."

Some individuals have been able to have their insulin requirement reduced or completely eliminated within a few weeks. These, of course, are spectacular cases. There are also insulin-taking diabetics who require a year or two to bring about a complete correction. The individual must be extremely cooperative. Attempts to correct diabetes <u>must be done under the supervision of a doctor.</u>

Dr. Eck says that those taking oral hypoglycemic agents for diabetics are the easiest cases to correct. Correcting those with juvenile diabetes is much more difficult ... unless the individual faithfully stays on the health program.

The MINERAL Approach To Illness
An Interview with Paul Eck

Dr. Eck believes there are _7_ mineral clues as to whether a person is developing cancer. The more of these clues they have the more severe their condition is. Here are the clues:

*1. <u>Calcium/Magnesium</u> ratio of <u>less than</u> 2 parts of calcium to 1 part of magnesium . . . is a cancer indicator.

*2. <u>Calcium/Magnesium</u> ratio of <u>over</u> 14 parts of calcium to 1 part of magnesium . . . is a cancer indicator.

*3. <u>Sodium/Potassium inversion.</u> Normally sodium is <u>25</u> in ratio to your potassium, which is <u>10</u>. This is a 2.5 to 1 sodium to potassium ratio. If the ratio inverts (goes <u>lower</u> than 1.5 to 1) this could be indicative of cancer, kidney disease, hypertension, infections, osteoarthritis, etc.!

*4. <u>Zinc/copper</u> ratio of <u>over</u> 16 parts of zinc to 1 part of copper . . . is a cancer indicator.

*5. <u>Zinc/copper</u> ratio of <u>less than</u> 4 parts of zinc to 1 part of copper . . . is a cancer indicator.

*6. <u>Copper</u> greater than 10 and less than 1.0 irregardless of ratio's . . . is a cancer indicator.

*7. <u>Iron</u> greater than 10 and less than 1.0 . . . is a cancer indicator.

Paul Eck believes that there are important interrelationships between minerals and vitamins. An excess of one mineral can cause an imbalance in another mineral in your body. Such imbalances can lead to illness. Here are some examples:

1. <u>MANGANESE</u>
Manganese can lower <u>magnesium</u> levels in the body. If your magnesium level is already low, the additional lowering by taking manganese can cause epileptic seizures and other neuro-muscular dysfunctions.

2. <u>CALCIUM</u>
Whenever you take large amounts of calcium, Eck states you will lose potassium. He says about 80% of the people in the United States suffer from a sluggish thyroid. This causes a high blood cholesterol, lack of incentive, fatigue. Eck says:

---

*These ratios figures are Paul Eck's testing figures. They are not standard ratio figures. What other testing laboratories for hair analysis may consider a normal ratio . . . Eck may consider not in the normal range.

> *Potassium is necessary for thyroxin, which is a hormone of the thyroid gland.*

Therefore, if one takes calcium causing a lowering in potassium he will have a lowering of thryoid function.

Calcium will also drive magnesium out of the body causing a high level of phosphorus to occur and make one prone to dental cavities.

3. Vitamin B$_1$

   Large amounts of Vitamin B$_1$ can over a period of time cause a <u>manganese</u> deficiency. Initially, the taking of Vitamin B$_1$ *(thiamine)* will give you a burst of energy. The excess of this B vitamin may also cause a <u>magnesium</u> deficiency. Both manganese and magnesium are important, Eck says, in blood sugar problems. Because of this manganese/magnesium dificiency, Eck believes, they can develop over 70 different diseases . . . including diabetes.

4. IRON

   Iron supplements can cause a copper deficiency. When too much iron is taken, Eck states, you can cause extremely high blood pressure, migraine headaches, and arthritis. Many arthritics have iron deposits in the joints of the body. Eck also reveals:

   > *Over 51% of all the cases of heart disease have been found to have iron pigment deposits in the cardiac cells of the heart . . . largely from taking too much iron or an inability to properly metabolize iron.[1]*

   To give iron to raise iron is to lower iron. This is true of every mineral. When you have an iron deficiency, you give manganese.

5. ZINC

   Zinc supplements can cause a copper deficiency resulting in a severe anemia. By causing a copper deficiency the following conditions may result—menstrual problems, prostrate disorders, allergies, arthritis and insomnia to name a few.

6. COPPER supplements can over a period of time result in a Vitamin C deficiency. Excessive copper can also cause a Vitamin B-1 and B-6 deficiency.

---

[1]Ibid.

The MINERAL Approach To Illness
An Interview with Paul Eck

Impotency and frigidity problems are intimately associated with mineral ratio imbalances caused by "stress," diabetes, hypothyroidism, adrenal insufficiency, etc.

The **seven** main indicators, from a hair analysis, of impotence in a male or frigidity in the female are:

1. A 3.3 to 1 or less of calcium to magnesium level indicates that the individual has sexual problems of impotence or frigidity. This inverted ratio is found particularly in diabetics.
2. Sodium/Potassium inversion. The normal ratio is 2.5 of sodium to 1 of potassium. If this is inverted (less than 1.8/1), it is an indicator of sexual problems.
3. Copper. A very high copper level is another indicator.
4. Zinc. Extremely low or high zincs can also indicate sexual dysfunction and be a cause of impotence or frigidity.
5. A Sodium/Magnesium ratio greater than   18/1.
6. A Sodium/Zinc ratio greater than   8/1.
7. A Calcium/Sodium ratio greater than   10/1.

In the problems of obesity (overweight), Dr. Eck breaks down individuals into broad categories such as:

Fast oxidation
Slow oxidation
Mixed oxidation

There are   3   different ways people metabolize their food. Dr. Eck refers to this as _Oxidation._ Oxidation is the use or burning of foods to produce energy on a cellular level. Regarding oxidation, Dr. Eck identifies the categories and suggests:

1. They are so fast
   they are breaking down their sugars very rapidly and they have a great increase in heat production as a result. They are the type of people who, when they eat, they perspire a lot. They are _"fast oxidizers."_ A _"fast oxidizer"_ is a person who has a hyperactive thyroid and hyperactive adrenal glands. They tend to have excessive energy levels due to the fast burning of foods, followed by exhaustion.

2. They are so <u>slow</u>

that they are metabolizing their foods very slowly. They are *"slow oxidizers."* They have a <u>hypo</u>active thyroid and <u>hypo</u>active adrenal glands. Slow oxidizer's energy levels are usually low. This can be due to a number of factors such as the body's inability to completely break down the foods consumed when a HCl (Hydrochloric acid) deficiency is present. Low thyroid and adrenal activity also contributes to slow oxidation as well as toxic metal accumulation and dietary habits.

3. They are <u>mixed</u> oxidizers

who may be fast in one glandular area and slow in another. They tend to have energy swings as well as mood swings. This is due to the *"seesaw"* effect from fluctuating into fast and slow oxidation.

Both the fast and slow oxidizers are handling their foods the wrong way.

The Pill Destroys Sex Life Of Women

Dr. Eck believes that the Pill has destroyed the sex life of at least 10 million women.

The Pill creates a false pregnancy. The taking of a birth control pill raises the copper levels in the body. This creates a mineral imbalance which lowers your thyroid function as well as adrenal activity.

When a person has a low thyroid activity (<u>hypo</u>thyroid), they don't have anywhere near the sex arousal . . . nor do they have a strong sex desire. They don't have the energy for it! Not only that, but the Pill brings with it menstrual period irregularities and menopausal disorders.

The male with <u>high</u> copper levels also develops a <u>**slow**</u> sexual arousal. Food that are high in copper include Brazil nuts, peanuts, sesame seeds, corn grits, broiled cod, baked flounder, broiled halibut, steamed lobster, pike and perch, ham, liver. <u>Oysters are extremely high in copper.</u> Just 1 cup of oysters (cooked, fried or raw) contains 59 milligrams of copper!

You also take copper into your body by drinking water coming through copper water pipes or cooking out of copper cookware.

Some women wear a copper IUD birth control device. Because the vagina is an acid medium . . . that acidity leaches the copper off the coil and it goes into your system. Dr. Eck states that:

> *It is estimated that there is enough copper*
> *eroded from a coil in one year*
> *to actually cause a person*
> *to become schizophrenic.*[1]

In a pregnant woman, the copper keeps building up during pregnancy. The fetus stores a large amount of copper that he gets from his mother's liver. This usually last the child for 12 years.

> *At the end of 12 years . . . if the child's copper level*
> *does not go down . . . you have females complaining of*
> *acne and adolescent problems, etc.*

If the mother cannot quickly unload the copper excess after pregnancy . . . she develops postpartum depression. Some women have become mentally unbalanced after giving birth. Paul Eck believes that copper excesses are the problem. Depending on the mineral imbalances of the individual, Eck uses either minerals or vitamins to unload the copper excesses. The hair analysis determines what supplements are needed.

What Results Can One Expect

Dr. Eck states that those who have a hair analysis and follow through on a personalized supplement program will experience symptomatic changes within two to three weeks. At least one year on supplements is needed to approach normalized mineral levels. Toxic metals and toxic minerals can be flushed out in about 6 months.

They may experience periodic worsening of their general condition depending upon their findings. As an example, if a person has rheumatoid arthritis, many times within the first two weeks there may be a marked reduction in pain. However, if the individual has

---

[1]Schizophrenia is *a major mental disorder typically characterized by a separation between the thought processes and the emotions . . . a distortion of reality accompanied by delusions and hallucinations.*

numerous heavy metal accumulation, the removal from tissues and joints of these toxic metals will trigger a temporary flare-up in their condition. This may occur several times throughout the program. Dr. Eck suggests that if this flare-up of symptoms becomes too severe, the individual should reduce or stop taking his supplements for a few days until the symptoms subside.

Permanents, tints, bleaching and coloring of hair does not make any significant changes in hair analysis mineral readings. Some shampoos and hair treatments do affect mineral levels, however.

Selsun Blue may cause an elevation in selenium levels.
Head and Shoulders or Breck may result in elevated zinc.
Grecian Formula or other darkening agents will many times result in elevated lead levels. Lead acetate is used in these products to blacken the hair.

Dr. Eck suggests that hair analysis retests should be done three months after the first test to check progress. If the individual is a *"mixed ozidizer"* or *"fast oxidizer,"* a retest is suggested in two months.

Dr. Eck says you cannot treat these people exactly the same as far as anything is concerned. You must take into consideration a broad classification of their oxidation types ... preparing a program on that premise. You cannot give any one mineral for an obesity problem or any other problem. Hair analysis will determine what minerals are deficient and what minerals are in excess.

Paul Eck is very sold on proper hair analysis. In fact he is so sold on the necessity for hair analysis that he would not suggest any mode of treatment for any condition ... to a physician ... until a hair analysis of the patient has been made.

Hair analysis is becoming more and more popular. And there are quite a few hair analysis laboratories throughout the United States. Not all agree with Dr. Paul Eck's approach. In fact, he may be considered a maverick in the field. But his laboratory in Phoenix is kept very busy. It could be a sign that his customers are getting excellent results from his recommendations![1]

---

[1] Dr. Paul Eck, Analytical Research Labs, Inc., 2338 West Royal Palm Road, Suite F, Phoenix, Arizona 85021

14

VITAMIN F AND THE PROSTATE

Lubricates Cells

Vitamin F is known as *unsaturated fatty acids*. It is a fat-soluble vitamin. Unsaturated fatty acids usually come in the form of liquid vegetable oils, while saturated fatty acids are usually found in solid animal fat.

Unsaturated fatty acids consist of:

    linoleic
    linolenic
    arachidonic

and they must be obtained from foods.

Wheat germ; seeds; natural golden vegetable oils, such as safflower, sunflower, soy and corn; and cod-liver oil contain lecithin and are the best sources of unsaturated fatty acids.[1]

Vitamin F (unsaturated fatty acids) help maintain resilience and lubrication of all cells and are essential for normal glandular activity. Men usually need five times more saturated fatty acids than women do. A balance of twice as much unsaturated fatty acids as saturated fatty acids in the daily diet is beneficial for health. About four or five tablespoons of vegetable oils per day (or via supplement) are needed to maintain this balance.

Vitamin E Aids Absorption

The greatest benefit is achieved with Vitamin F if Vitamin E is also taken along with it at mealtimes. This ensures the best absorption. Fatty acids are found in the tissues of the prostate gland.

In one test, 19 cases of prostate gland disorders were treated with unsaturated fatty acids. All 19 had a lessening of residual urine (urine that cannot be released from the bladder due to pressure from the enlarged prostate gland).

There was also a decrease in leg pains, fatigue, kidney disorders and excessive urination at night.

The seeds which have the highest concentrate of unsaturated fatty acids are:

Sunflower seeds
Pumpkin seeds

OTHER NON-SURGICAL METHODS

Homeopathic Methods

Homeopathy (*like* + *disease*) assumes that medicines which cure disease produce similar symptoms in the healthy. The drugs used are given in extremely small doses.

Homeopathy school of medicine was founded by Dr. S. C. F. Hahnemann in 1796 in Philadelphia. There is a hospital in Philadelphia today called Hahnemann although it now practices standard medical procedures.

They have about 15 different drug tinctures for a variety of prostate symptoms. As an example, _Aconite_ is for Prostatitis . . . where there is a great urging to urinate and burning pain during urination. The various formulas are sold in health food stores.

Other homeopathic prostate drugs include: Apis, Cuasticum, Chimaphila, Conium mac, Pareira brava, Pulsatilla and Sabal serrulata.

FASTING BRINGS IMPROVEMENT

Fasting

Dr. Herbert Shelton and his staff conduct a supervised fasting clinic in Texas. They state that by fasting and following a natural hygienic system enlarged prostate glands were reduced to normal size in about 7 days following their program. Most cases take longer, however. The improvement is generally not permanent since the individual goes back to old eating and living habits.

UNUSUAL WHEAT GRASS CLAIMS

Wheat Grass Therapy

Anne Wigmore is perhaps the originator of the Wheat Grass therapy program. This originates in Boston, Massachusetts.

Anne Wigmore _first_ seeks to rebuild the body by providing a simple diet at her retreat which includes raw foods and vitamin and mineral therapy. _Each guest also drinks_ three 3-ounce drinks of freshly squeezed out _wheat grass juice_ each day between meals.

Rectal Implant Promising

Also, at least three times a day, the guest must *"implant"* in his rectum at least a half glass of freshly squeezed out wheat grass juice. To do this he props his abdomen up on pillows or a slant board so that the liquid can come as close as possible to the prostate gland and be partially absorbed through the tissues.

Anne Wigmore states:

> *We have never had an unfortunate*
> *with prostate trouble*
> *whether chronic or acute*
> *that did not respond favorably*
> *to this three-ply method.*
>
> *In many, many instances,*
> *operations that had been scheduled,*
> *were abandoned by the medical doctors*
> *who had heretofore believed*
> *that they were vitally necessary.*[1]

RESTORING IMPAIRED NERVE FUNCTION

Chiropractic Treatment

The chiropractor seeks to correct spinal subluxations so that the body can correct its own ailments. A spinal column out of adjustment may impinge and restrict the motor and sensory nerve supply to various structures of the body including the prostate. A chiropractic adjustment is considered by many an important first step to healing of the prostate.

[1]John D. Kirschmann, Nutrition Almanac (New York: McGraw-Hill Book Company) 1975, p. 55.

A HUMOROUS PHILOSOPHY

The Tide Turns!

The late John H. Tobe, who was a colorful and energetic advocate of natural health methods penned this poem at the beginning of his book, Your Prostate:

> He who with swift, unerring hand,
> Has oft removed a prostate gland,
> Has reaped the harvest he has sown . . .
> He's having trouble with his own!

[1]John H. Tobe, Your Prostate: Treatment and Prevention (St. Catharines, Ontario, Canada: Provoker Press) 1968, p. 338.

FOR YOUR <u>LIFE</u> . . . KEEP INFORMED!

Now available! A quarterly Total Health Guide Newsletter to keep you up-to-date on the <u>very latest</u> of Medical/Nutritional Data! You owe it to yourself and to your loved ones . . . to be fully informed! Now! At last! You can have the <u>most current</u> information on diseases and their treatment . . . even before it is available to the general public! The information you receive may help save your life . . . or the life of a loved one!

<u>TWO</u> WAYS TO SUBSCRIBE

1. <u>Total Health Guide Newsletter</u>

Quarterly, for one year we will send you the 8-page Newsletter containing all the latest data on the major diseases. The Newsletter will present an unbiased report on both the Medical and Nutritional discoveries plus reports on their effectiveness and availability.

One Year: $25

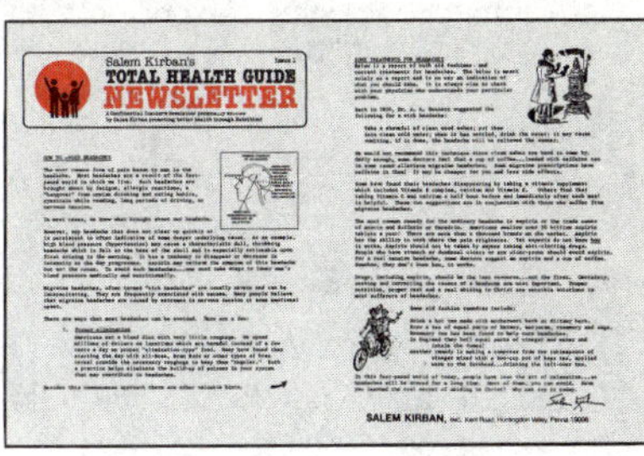

2. Total Health Guide Newsletter
Plus
PERSONALIZED TYPEWRITTEN UPDATE

You will receive the quarterly 8-page Newsletter which reports the latest in Medical and Nutritional approaches to disease.

Plus! You will also receive a <u>TYPEWRITTEN REPORT</u> on the <u>specific disease in which you are personally interested.</u> This TYPEWRITTEN REPORT will be mailed to you within 3 weeks after you subscribe.

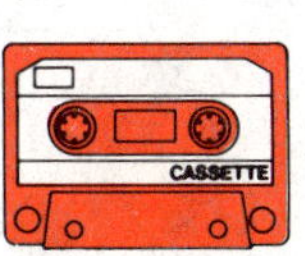

- You will also receive a <u>RING BINDER</u> to hold the Newsletters and Report. It will also contain a special unit to hold cassettes.

- Plus you will be sent the <u>cassette</u> . . .
  BALANCING YOUR EMOTIONS
  by Dr. Jonas Miller.

One Year: $50

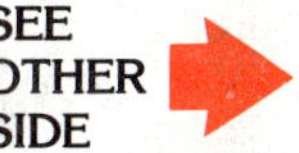

SEE OTHER SIDE →

SALEM KIRBAN, Inc., Kent Road, Huntingdon Valley, Pennsylvania 19006

YES! I want to keep informed! Send me the Health Information Service I have checked below. My check is enclosed.

☐ 1 Year / $25
Total Health Newsletter

☐ 1 Year / $50 *(Fill in other side)*
Total Health Newsletter
Typewritten Health Report
(Includes Ring Binder/Cassette)

Mr./Mrs./Miss ________________________ (Please PRINT)

Address ________________________

City ________________ State ______ ZIP ______

REQUEST For Personalized TYPEWRITTEN HEALTH UPDATE

If you are subscribing for Medical/Nutritional Health Information for One Year at $50, you are entitled to a Typewritten Health Update on one disease.

It is important you understand that we neither diagnose or prescribe. Therefore we **cannot** make personal recommendations to you. Only your physician can do this. What we do provide you is the very latest in both Medical and Nutritional information on the disease in which you are interested.

Each month we go through hundreds of publications, books and listen to both medical and nutritional seminar cassettes. We cull from all of this the data that is essential to the particular disease in which you are interested.

We would be happy to answer specific questions in this TYPEWRITTEN HEALTH UPDATE providing they are not in the realm of diagnosing or prescribing.

DISEASE I want Data on____

MY QUESTIONS I particularly would like answered: *(Please PRINT)*

1. ____

____

____

2. ____

____

____

3 ____

____

____

4. ____

____

____

FILL IN
RESPONSE FORM
ON
REVERSE SIDE
AND
MAIL WITH YOUR CHECK

Use this ORDER FORM to order additional copies of

The MEDICAL Approach Versus NUTRITIONAL Approach To PROSTATE PROBLEMS
by Salem Kirban

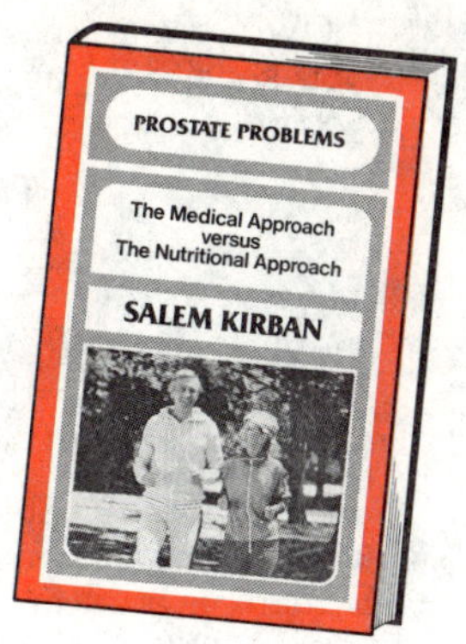

Your loved ones and friends will find this book invaluable! Why not give this excellent book to those who want honest answers to their problems.

QUANTITY PRICES:

1 copy: $5.00

3 copies: $12 (You save $3)
5 copies: $20 (You save $5)

ORDER FORM

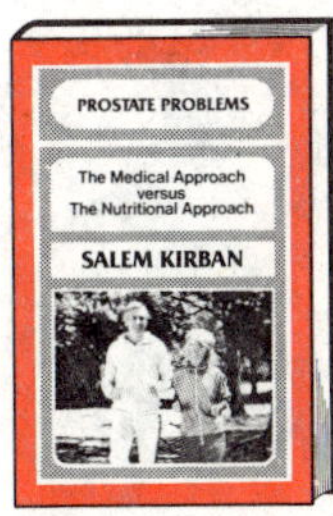

Salem Kirban, Inc.
Kent Road
Huntingdon Valley, Pennsylvania 19006

Enclosed find $ _______ (plus $1 postage) for _______ copies of

The MEDICAL Approach Versus The NUTRITIONAL Approach to PROSTATE PROBLEMS by Salem Kirban

Name____
    Mr./Mrs./Miss   (Please PRINT)

Street_______________________________________

City____

State__________________________ Zip Code__________________

NOW! . . . You can make intelligent, life-changing decisions when you know **both approaches** to correcting ailments that plague you or your loved ones!

THE MEDICAL APPROACH
versus
THE NUTRITIONAL APPROACH

NEVER BEFORE . . . in one book . . . has an unbiased comparison been outlined, clearly, simply, showing both the Medical approach versus the Nutritional approach to major diseases!

At last! Sixteen books are now available! Each book defines the disease in words you can understand plus graphic pictures. The symptoms are also outlined.

Each book shows how medical doctors approach the examination of the patient, what tests they conduct, what drugs they recommend (and their side effects), the type of surgery followed and what their prediction is regarding the course of the disease and the probability of recovery (termed, *prognosis*).

In the same book, you will also read the Nutritional approach to the same disease; what natural therapy has been used through the years, what results have been achieved and what the prognosis is using nature's way.

Save by buying several books. Give to loved ones. You may be giving a gift of LIFE! **Each book is $5.**

KIDNEY DISEASE

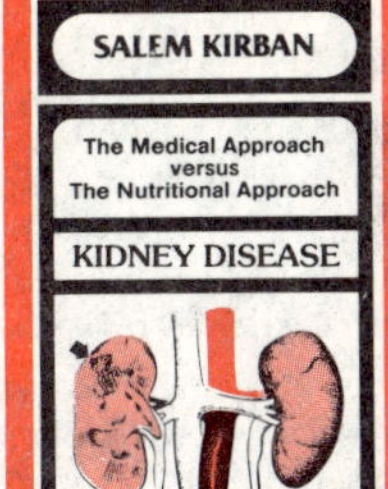

(9)

by Salem Kirban

What is the medical approach to kidney disease? What are some of the problems that can develop if the disease is not nipped in the bud? What are the side effects of the drugs prescribed?

Is meat harmful? What type of diet is beneficial? Is a supervised fast recommended? How long? What common, ordinary foods and juices have proven beneficial? What vitamins and minerals help? What about herbs?

EYESIGHT

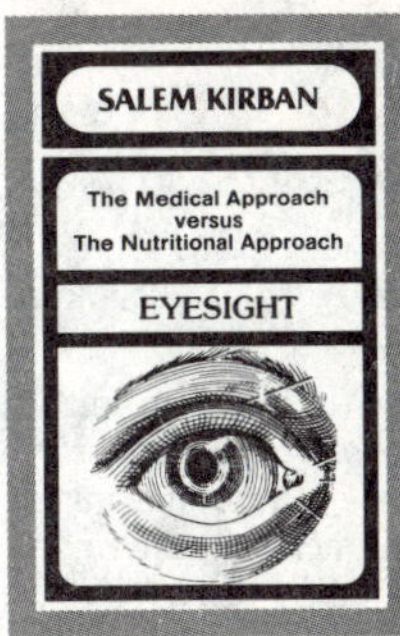

(10)

by Salem Kirban

Are glasses the answer to failing eyesight? Is the medical approach to Cataracts the only solution? What do nutritionists recommend?

What eye exercises may prove beneficial for my eyes? Can I throw away my glasses? Is poor eyesight an indication of other growing physical problems? Can diet correct my poor eyesight? What juices may prove beneficial? What combination of vitamins and minerals should I take?

IMPOTENCE/ FRIGIDITY

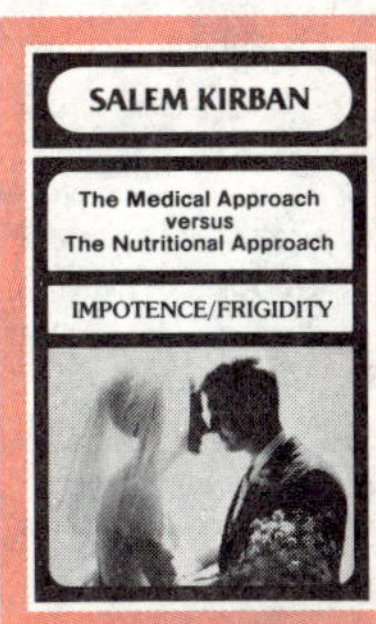

(11)

by Salem Kirban

Impotence is the incapacity of the male to have sexual union. Frigidity is the incapacity of the female for sexual response. Both of these problems are growing because of today's stressful lifestyle! They lead to other trials!

What is the medical approach to these problems? How successful are they? What is the nutritional approach? What type of diet is recommended? Do juices help? Are herbs beneficial? Much more!

COLITIS/CROHN'S DISEASE

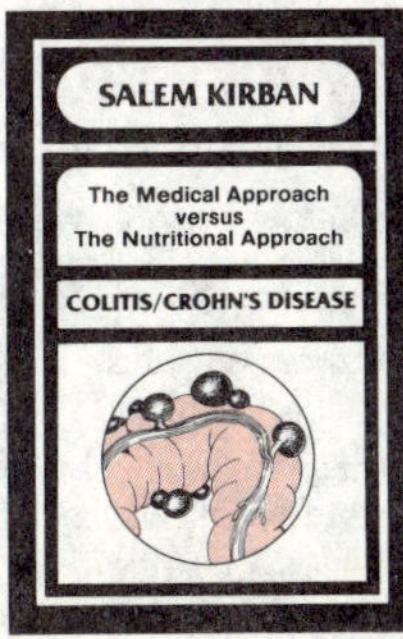

(12)

by Salem Kirban

What causes Colitis? What drugs do doctors recommend? What are the side effects: How successful is surgery? What is the nutritional approach to Colitis? What foods are beneficial? What about juices and vitamins?

What is Crohn's Disease? What are the symptoms? Why does it recur? What is the medical approach to the problem? What is the nutritional approach? Can juices and vitamins correct the cause?

Quantity	Description	Price	Total

The MEDICAL APPROACH Versus The NUTRITIONAL APPROACH Series

	1 Arthritis	$ 5.00	
	2 Cancer	5.00	
	3 Heart Disease	5.00	
	4 High Blood Pressure	5.00	
	5 Diabetes	5.00	
	6 Bowel Problems	5.00	
	7 Prostate Problems	5.00	
	8 Ulcers	5.00	
	9 Kidney Disease	5.00	
	10 Eyesight	5.00	
	11 Impotence and Frigidity	5.00	
	12 Colitis/Crohn's Disease	5.00	
	13 How To Be Young Again	5.00	
	14 Obesity	5.00	
	15 Headaches	5.00	
	16 Hypoglycemia	5.00	
	All 16 Health Books *(Save $30)*	**$50.00**	

Single Book	$5	All 16 Books	$50*
Any 3 Books	$12	(*You save $30)	

Other SALEM KIRBAN HEALTH BOOKS

Unlocking Your Bowels For Better Health	4.95	
How Juices Restore Health Naturally	4.95	
How To Eat Your Way Back To Vibrant Health	4.95	
How To Keep Healthy & Happy By Fasting	4.95	
The Getting Back To Nature Diet	4.95	
How To Win Over IMPOTENCE/FRIGIDITY	6.95	
(Expanded Version with Full Color Section)		

Total for Books _______

Shipping & Handling _______

Total Enclosed $ _______

(We do NOT invoice. Check must accompany order, please.)

When using Credit Card, show number in space below.

☐ Check enclosed

☐ Master Charge

☐ VISA

When Using MasterCard Also Give Interbank No. (Just above your name on card)

Card Expires | Month | Year

***POSTAGE & HANDLING** Use the easy chart to figure postage, shipping and handling charges. Send correct amount and avoid delay.

TOTAL FOR BOOKS	Up to 5.00	5.01-10.00	10.01-20.00	20.01-35.00	Over 35.00
DELIVERY CHARGE	1.50	2.00	2.50	2.95	NO CHARGE

SHIP TO _______________________________
Mr./Mrs./Miss   (Please PRINT)

Address _______________________________

City _______________________ State ________ ZIP __________

SALEM KIRBAN, Inc./Kent Road, Huntingdon Valley, Pennsylvania 19006